The Ultimate Alkaline Guide to Smoothies for Beginners

Easy and Fast Recipes for Incredibly Healthy and Delicious Smoothies

I0134861

Bella Francis

contained within this document, including, but not limited to, — errors, omissions, or inaccuracies.

Table of contents

Raisins – Plume Smoothie (Rps)

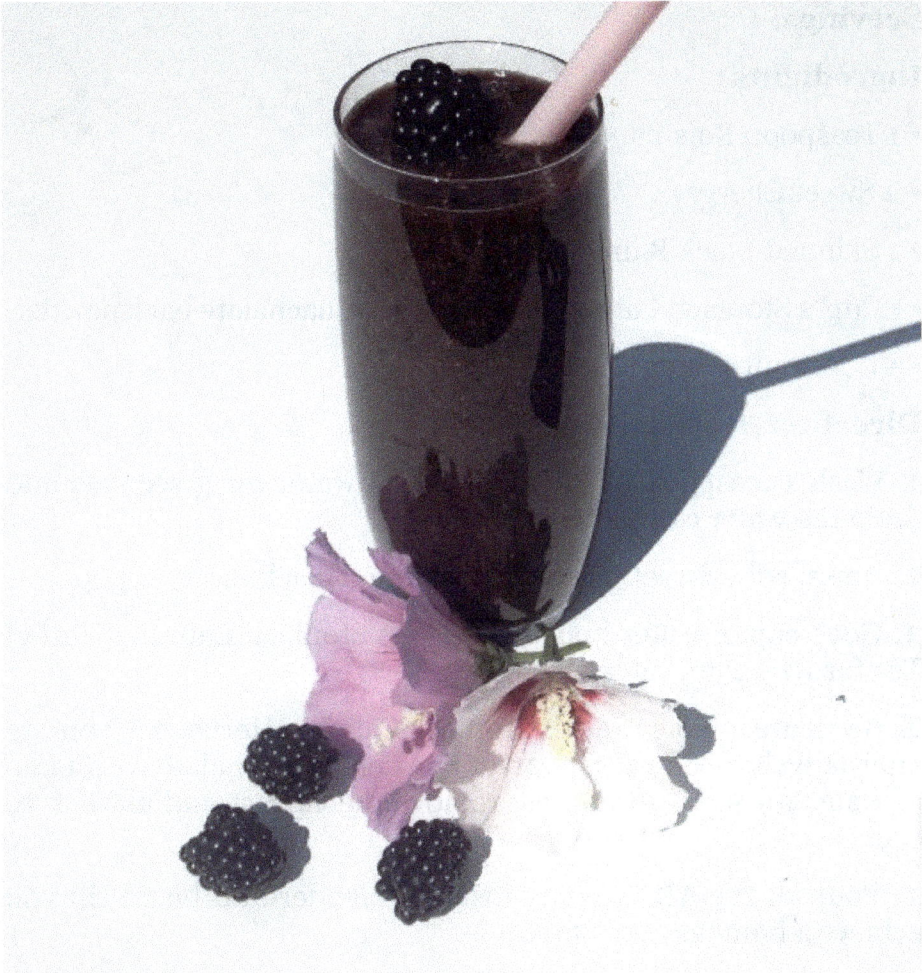

Preparation Time: 10 minutes

Cooking Time: 0 minutes

Servings: 1

Ingredients :

- 1 Teaspoon Raisins

- 2 Sweet Cherry

- 1 Skinned Black Plume

- 1 Cup 's Stomach Calming Herbal Tea/ Cuachalate back powder,

- ¼ Coconut Water

Directions:

1. Flash 1 teaspoon of Raisin in warm water for 5 seconds and drain the water completely.

2. Rinse, cube Sweet Cherry and skinned black Plum

3. Get 1 cup of water boiled; put ¾ 's Stomach Calming Herbal Tea for 10 – 15minutes.

4. If you are unable to get 's Stomach Calming Herbal tea, you can alternatively, cook 1 teaspoon of powdered Cuachalate with 1 cup of water for 5 – 10 minutes, remove the extract and allow it to cool.

5. Pour all the ARPS items inside a blender and blend till you achieve a homogenous smoothie.

6. It is now okay, for you to enjoy the inevitable detox smoothie.

Nutrition:

Calories: 150

Fat: 1.2 g

Carbohydrates: 79 g

Protein: 3.1 g

Nori Clove Smoothies (Ncs)

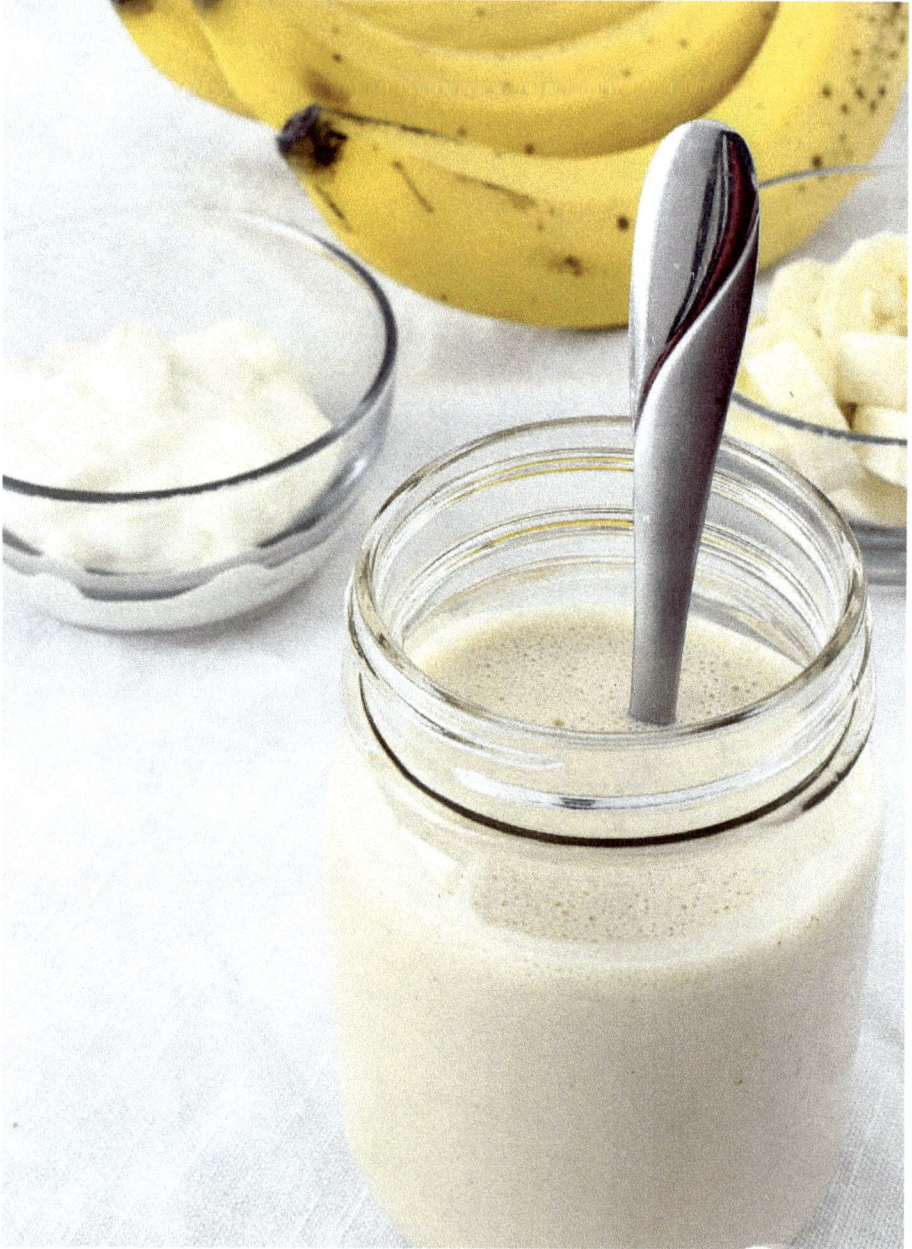

Preparation Time: 10 minutes

Cooking Time: 0 minutes

Servings: 1

Ingredients :

- ¼ Cup Fresh Nori

- 1 Cup Cubed Banana

- 1 Teaspoon Diced Onion or ¼ Teaspoon Powdered Onion

- ½ Teaspoon Clove

- 1 Cup Energy Booster

- 1 Tablespoon Agave Syrup

Directions:

1. Rinse ANCS Items with clean water.

2. Finely chop the onion to take one teaspoon and cut fresh Nori

3. Boil 1½ teaspoon with 2 cups of water, remove the particle, allow to cool, measure 1 cup of the tea extract

4. Pour all the items inside a blender with the tea extract and blend to achieve homogenous smoothies.

5. Transfer into a clean cup and have a nice time with a lovely body detox and energizer.

Nutrition:

Calories: 78

Fat: 2.3 g

Carbohydrates: 5 g

Protein: 6 g

Brazil Lettuce Smoothies (Bls)

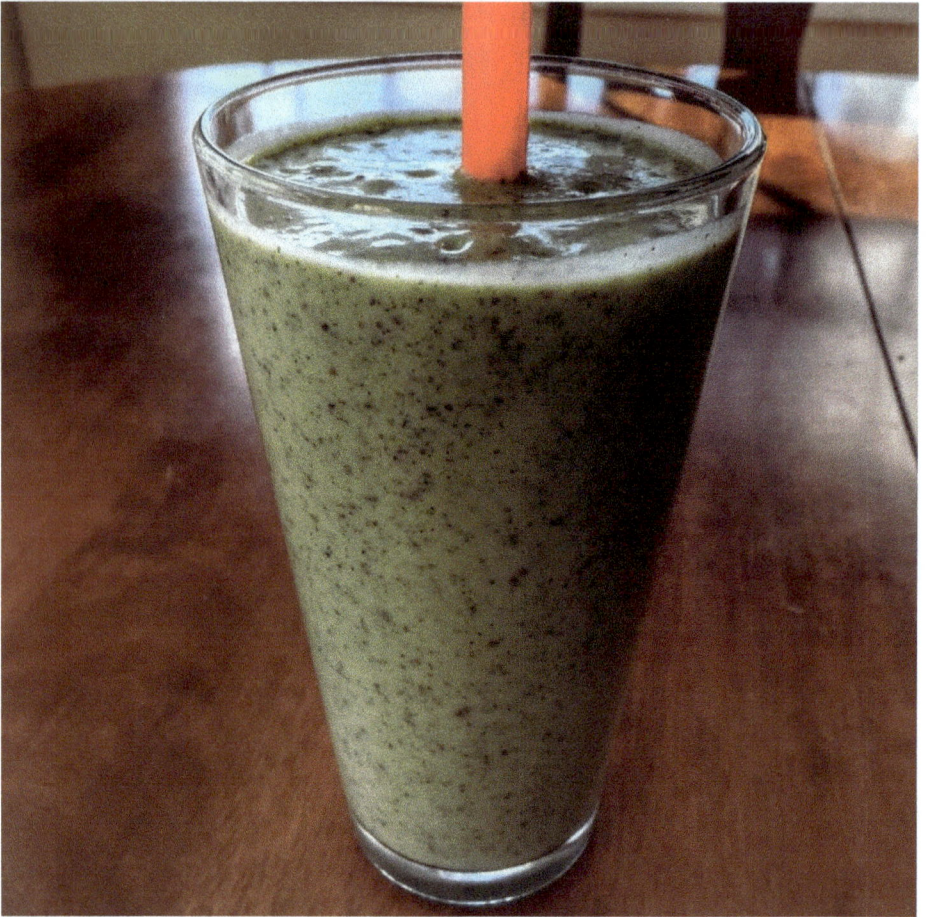

Preparation Time: 10 minutes

Cooking Time: 0 minutes

Servings: 1

Ingredients :

- 1 Cup Raspberries
- ½ Handful Romaine Lettuce
- ½ Cup Homemade Walnut Milk
- 2 Brazil Nuts
- ½ Large Grape with Seed
- 1 Cup Soft jelly Coconut Water
- Date Sugar to Taste

Directions:

1. In a clean bowl rinse the vegetable with clean water.

2. Chop the Romaine Lettuce and cubed Raspberries and add other items into the blender and blend to achieve homogenous smoothies.

3. Serve your delicious medicinal detox.

Nutrition:

Calories: 168

Fat: 4.5 g

Carbohydrates: 31.3 g

Sugar: 19.2 g

Protein: 3.6 g

Apple – Banana Smoothie (Abs)

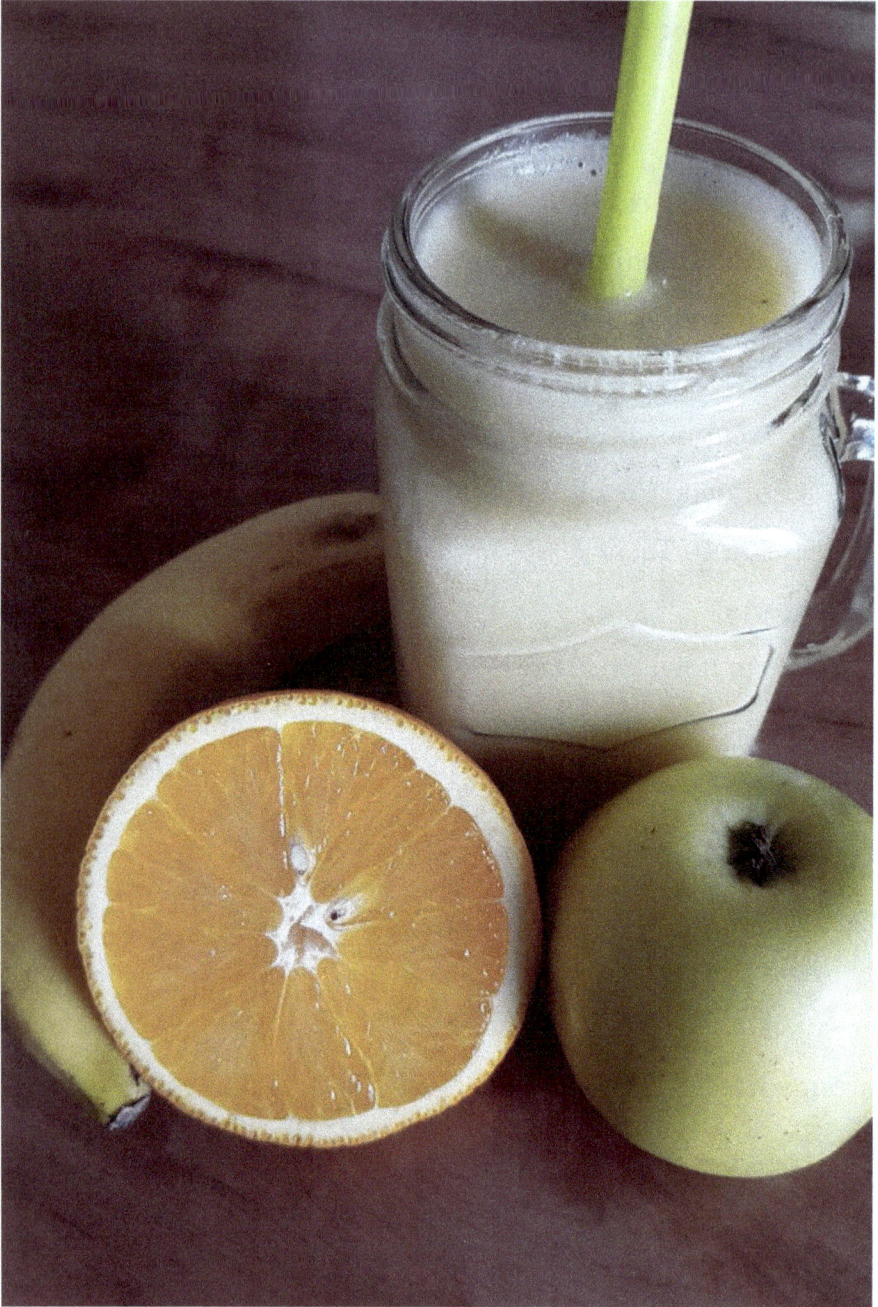

Preparation Time: 10 minutes

Cooking Time: 0 minutes

Servings: 1

Ingredients :

• I Cup Cubed Apple

• ½ Burro Banana

• ½ Cup Cubed Mango

• ½ Cup Cubed Watermelon

• ½ Teaspoon Powdered Onion

• 3 Tablespoon Key Lime Juice

• Date Sugar to Taste (If you like)

Directions:

1. In a clean bowl rinse the vegetable with clean water.

2. Cubed Banana, Apple, Mango, Watermelon and add other items into the blender and blend to achieve homogenous smoothies.

3. Serve your delicious medicinal detox.

4. Alternatively, you can add one tablespoon of finely dices raw red Onion if powdered Onion is not available.

Nutrition:

Calories: 99

Fat: 0.3g

Carbohydrates: 23 grams

Protein: 1.1 g

Ginger – Pear Smoothie (Gps)

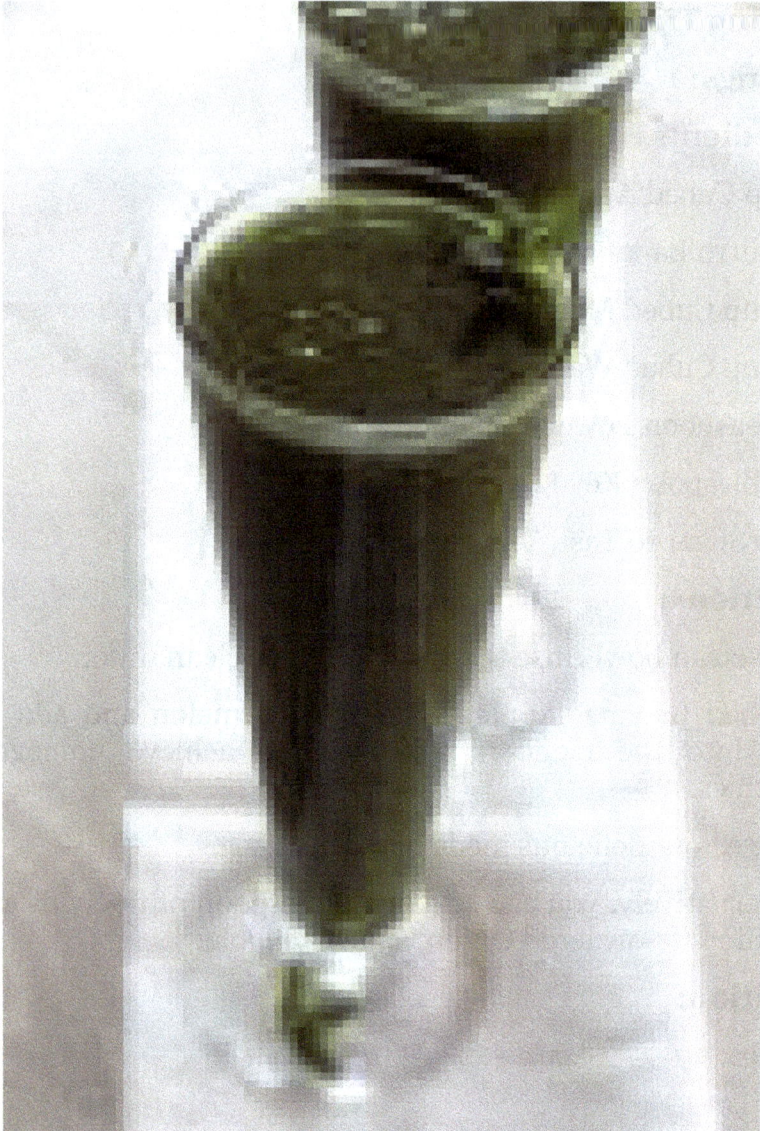

Preparation Time: 10 minutes

Cooking Time: 0 minutes

Servings: 1

Ingredients :

- 1 Big Pear with Seed and Cured
- ½ Avocado
- ¼ Handful Watercress
- ½ Sour Orange
- ½ Cup Ginger Tea
- ½ Cup Coconut Water
- ¼ Cup Spring Water
- 2 Tablespoon Agave Syrup
- Date Sugar to satisfaction

Directions:

1. Firstly boil 1 cup of Ginger Tea, cover the cup and allow it cool to room temperature.

2. Pour all the AGPS Items into your clean blender and homogenize them to smooth fluid.

3. You have just prepared yourself a wonderful Detox Romaine Smoothie.

Nutrition:

Calories: 101

Protein: 1 g

Carbs: 27 g

Fiber: 6 g

Cantaloupe – Amaranth Smoothie (Cas)

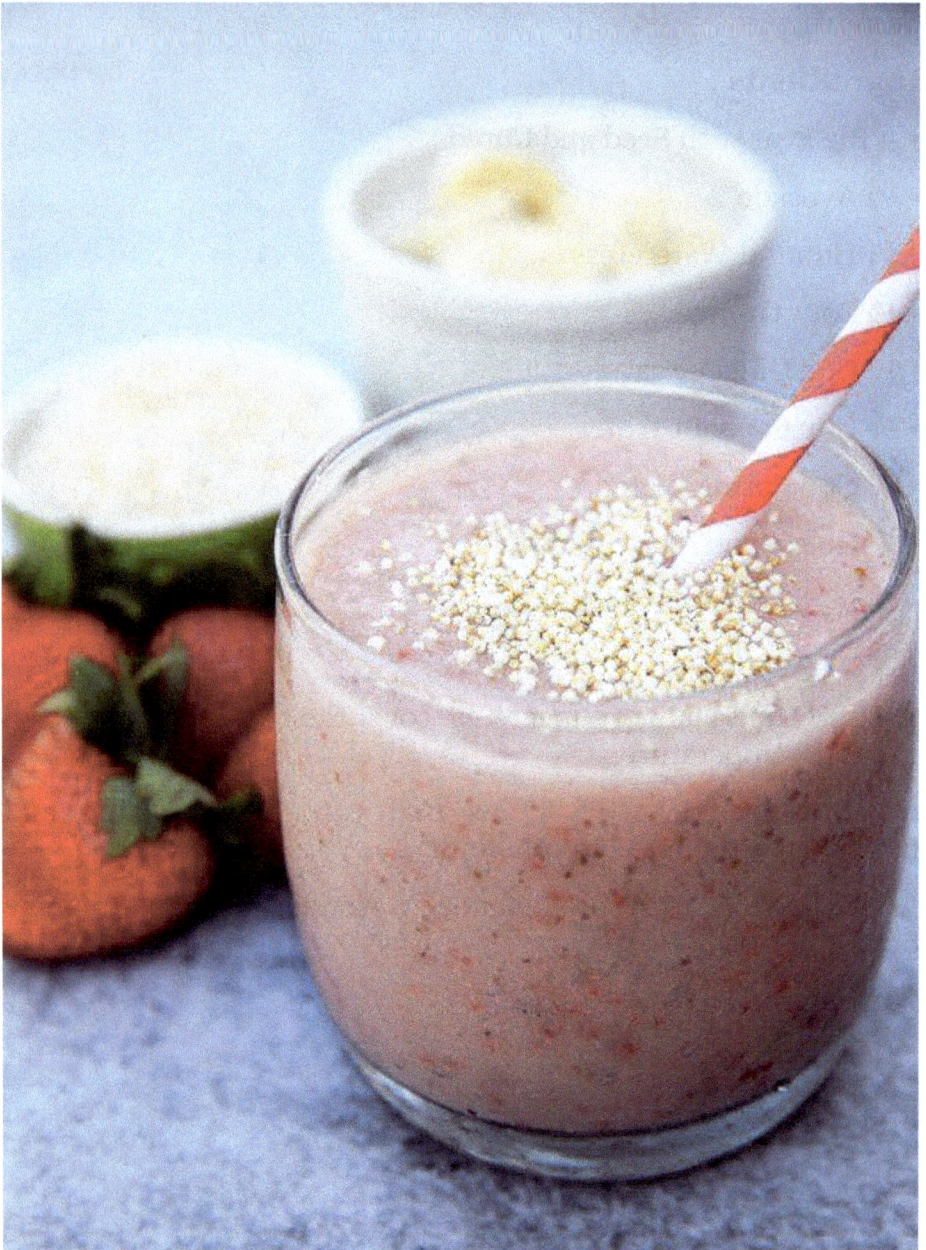

Preparation Time: 10 minutes

Cooking Time: 0 minutes

Servings: 1

Ingredients :

- ½ Cup Cubed Cantaloupe
- ¼ Handful Green Amaranth
- ½ Cup Homemade Hemp Milk
- ¼ Teaspoon 's Bromide Plus Powder
- 1 Cup Coconut Water
- 1 Teaspoon Agave Syrup

Directions:

1. You will have to rinse all the ACAS items with clean water.

2. Chop green Amaranth, cubed Cantaloupe, transfer all into a blender and blend to achieve homogenous smoothie.

3. Pour into a clean cup; add Agave syrup and homemade Hemp Milk.

4. Stir them together and drink.

Nutrition:

Calories: 55

Fiber: 1.5 g

Carbohydrates: 8 mg

Garbanzo Squash Smoothie (Gss)

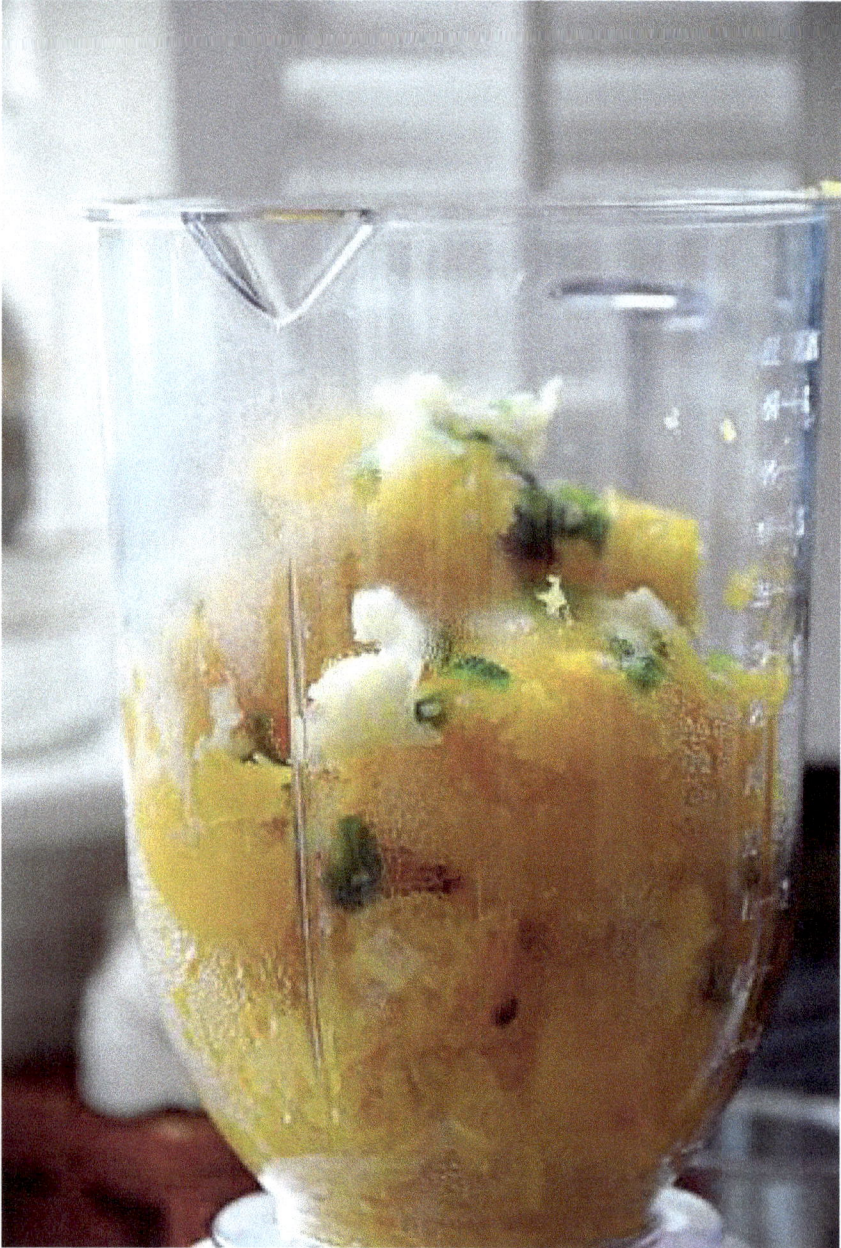

Preparation Time: 10 minutes

Cooking Time: 0 minutes

Servings: 1

Ingredients :

• 1 Large Cubed Apple

• 1 Fresh Tomatoes

• 1 Tablespoon Finely Chopped Fresh Onion or ¼ Teaspoon Powdered Onion

• ¼ Cup Boiled Garbanzo Bean

• ½ Cup Coconut Milk

• ¼ Cubed Mexican Squash Chayote

• 1 Cup Energy Booster Tea

Directions:

1. You will need to rinse the AGSS items with clean water.

2. Boil 1½ 's Energy Booster Tea with 2 cups of clean water. Filter the extract, measure 1 cup and allow it to cool.

3. Cook Garbanzo Bean, drain the water and allow it to cool.

4. Pour all the AGSS items into a high-speed blender and blend to achieve homogenous smoothie.

5. You may add Date Sugar.

6. Serve your amazing smoothie and drink.

Nutrition:

Calories: 82

Carbs: 22 g

Protein: 2 g

Fiber: 7 g

Strawberry – Orange Smoothies (Sos)

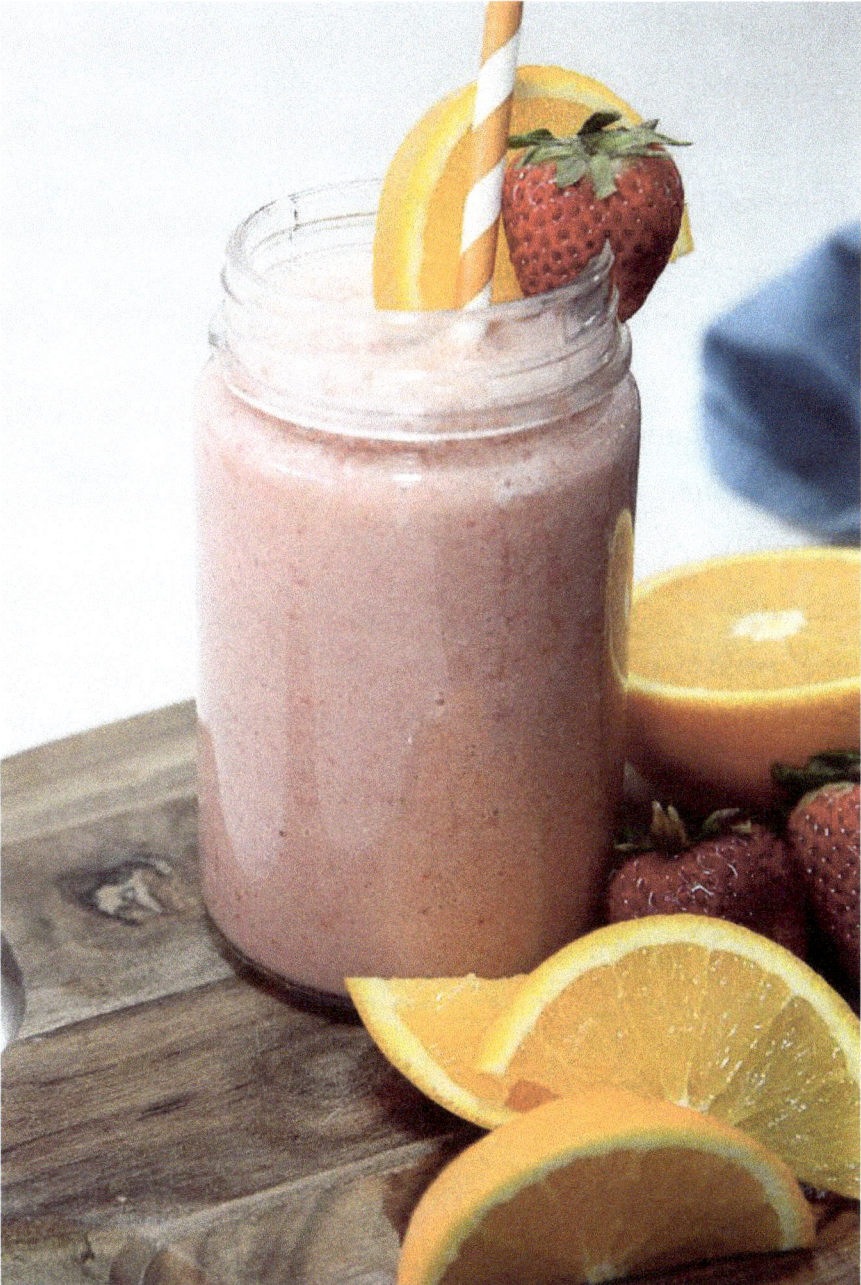

Preparation Time: 10 minutes

Cooking Time: 0 minutes

Servings: 1

Ingredients :

• 1 Cup Diced Strawberries

• 1 Removed Back of Seville Orange

• ¼ Cup Cubed Cucumber

• ¼ Cup Romaine Lettuce

• ½ Kelp

• ½ Burro Banana

• 1 Cup Soft Jelly Coconut Water

• ½ Cup Water

• Date Sugar.

Directions:

1. Use clean water to rinse all the vegetable items of ASOS into a clean bowl.

2. Chop Romaine Lettuce; dice Strawberry, Cucumber, and Banana; remove the back of Seville Orange and divide into four.

3. Transfer all the ASOS items inside a clean blender and blend to achieve a homogenous smoothie.

4. Pour into a clean big cup and fortify your body with a palatable detox.

Nutrition:

Calories 298

Calories from Fat 9

Fat 1g

Cholesterol 2mg

Sodium 73mg

Potassium 998mg

Carbohydrates 68g

Fiber 7g

Sugar 50g

Tamarind – Pear Smoothie (Tps)

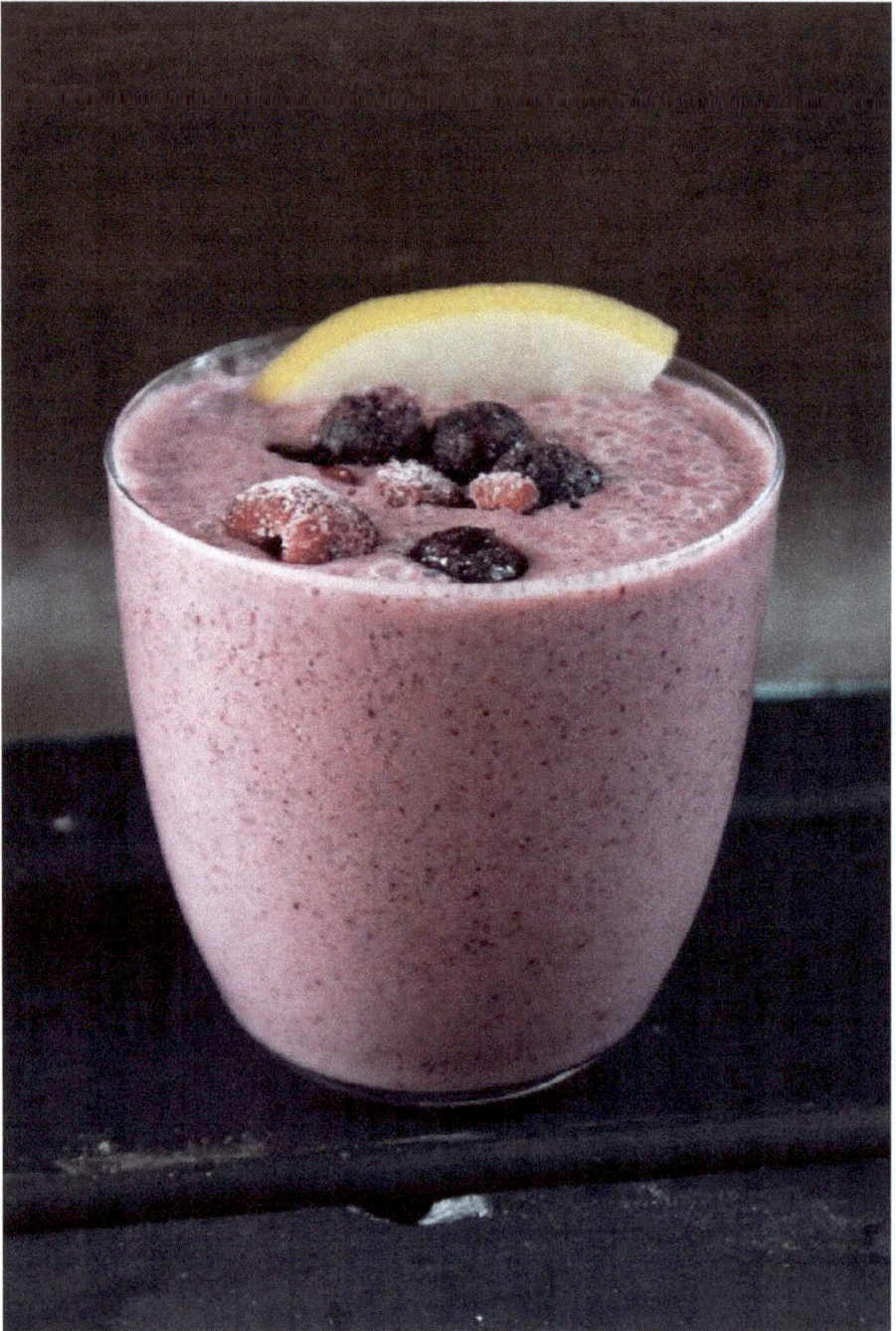

Preparation Time: 10 minutes

Cooking Time: 0 minutes

Servings: 1

Ingredients :

- ½ Burro Banana
- ½ Cup Watermelon
- 1 Raspberries
- 1 Prickly Pear
- 1 Grape with Seed
- 3 Tamarind
- ½ Medium Cucumber
- 1 Cup Coconut Water
- ½ Cup Distilled Water

Directions:

1. Use clean water to rinse all the ATPS items.

2. Remove the pod of Tamarind and collect the edible part around the seed into a container.

3. If you must use the seeds then you have to boil the seed for 15mins and add to the Tamarind edible part in the container.

4. Cubed all other vegetable fruits and transfer all the items into a high-speed blender and blend to achieve homogenous smoothie.

Nutrition:

Calories: 199

Carbohydrates: 47 g

Fat: 1g

Protein: 6g

Currant Elderberry Smoothie (Ces)

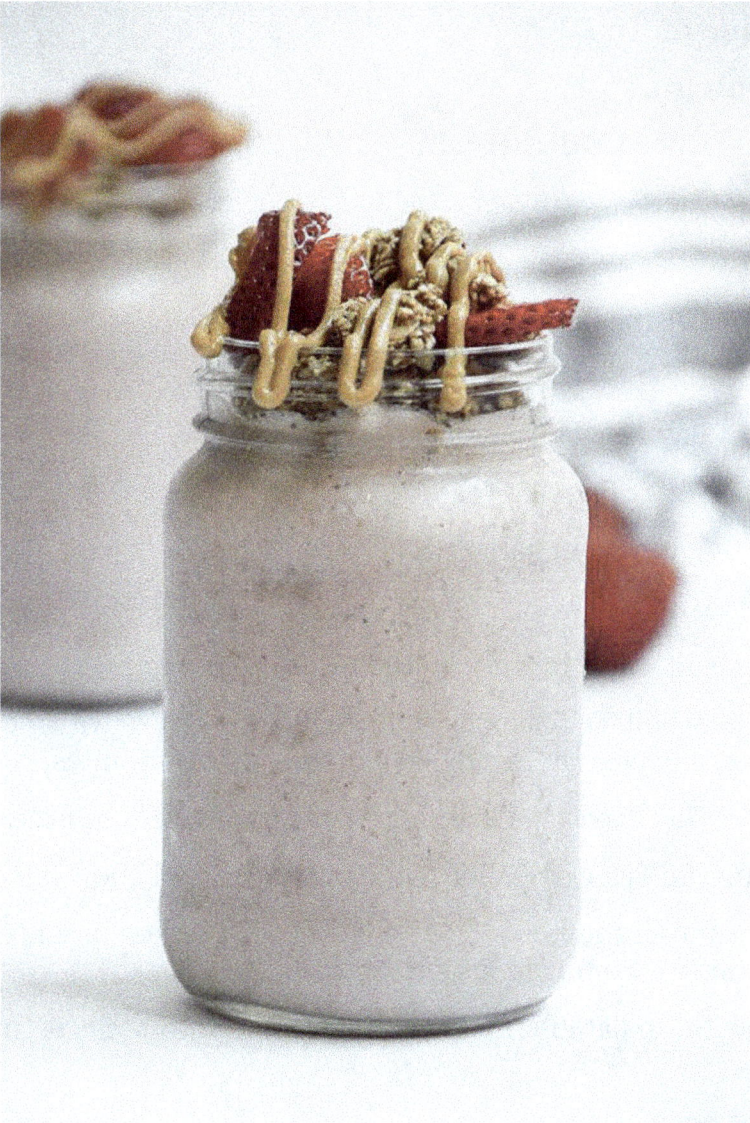

Preparation Time: 10 minutes

Cooking Time: 0 minutes

Servings: 1

Ingredients :

• ¼ Cup Cubed Elderberry

• 1 Sour Cherry

• 2 Currant

• 1 Cubed Burro Banana

• 1 Fig

• 1Cup 4 Bay Leaves Tea

• 1 Cup Energy Booster Tea

• Date Sugar to your satisfaction

Directions:

1. Use clean water to rinse all the ACES items

2. Initially boil ¾ Teaspoon of Energy Booster Tea with 2 cups of water on a heat source and allow boiling for 10 minutes.

3. Add 4 Bay leaves and boil together for another 4minutes.

4. Drain the Tea extract into a clean big cup and allow it to cool.

5. Transfer all the items into a high-speed blender and blend till you achieve a homogenous smoothie.

6. Pour the palatable medicinal smoothie into a clean cup and drink.

Nutrition:

Calories: 63

Fat: 0.22g

Sodium: 1.1mg

Carbohydrates: 15.5g

Fiber: 4.8g

Sugars: 8.25g

Protein: 1.6g

Sweet Dream Strawberry Smoothie

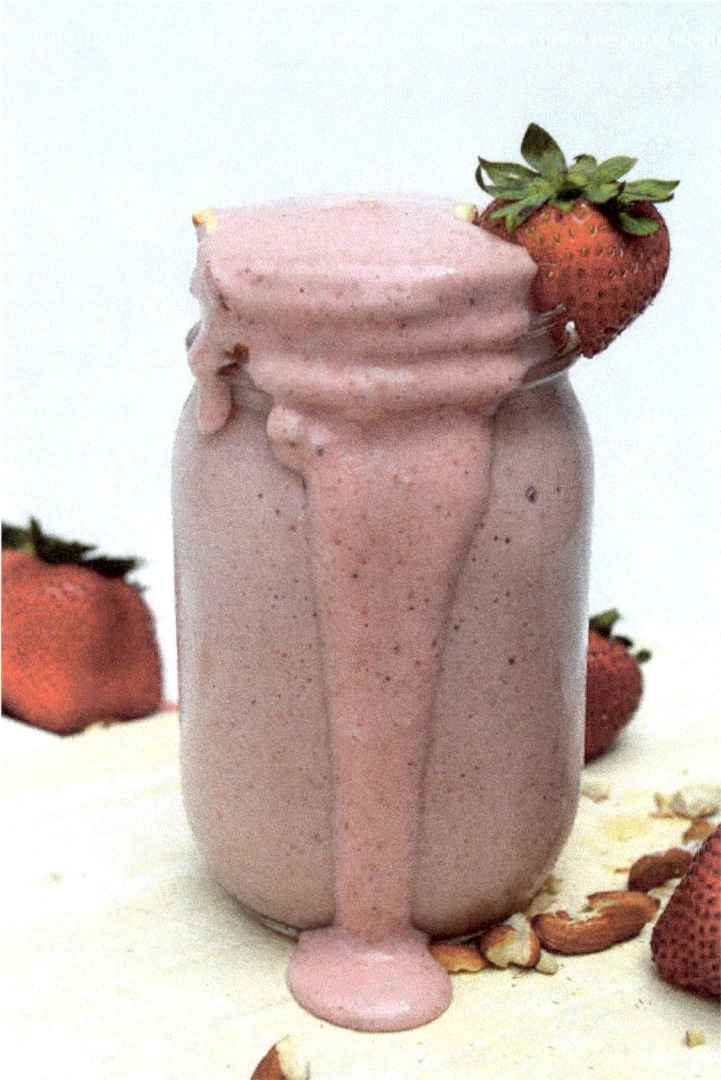

Preparation Time: 1 5 minutes

Cooking Time: 0

Servings: 1

Ingredients :

• 5 Strawberries

• 3 Dates – Pits eliminated

• 2 Burro Bananas or small bananas

• Spring Water for 32 fluid ounce of smoothie

Directions:

1. Strip off skin of the bananas.

2. Wash the dates and strawberries.

3. Include bananas, dates, and strawberries to a blender container.

4. Include a couple of water and blend.

5. Keep on including adequate water to persuade up to be 32 oz. of smoothie.

Nutrition:

Calories: 282

Fat: 11g

Carbohydrates: 4g

Protein: 7g

Alkaline Green Ginger And Banana Cleansing Smoothie

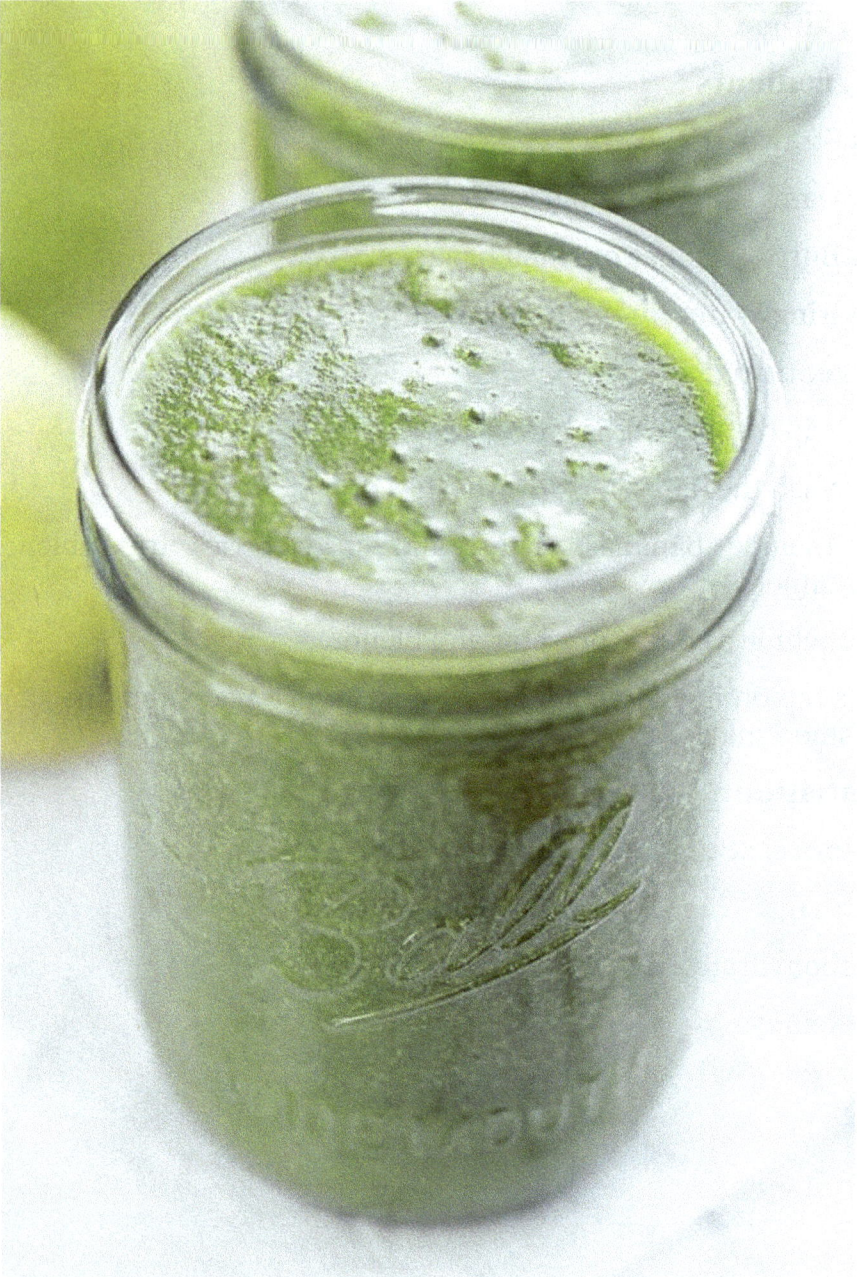

Preparation Time: 15 minutes

Cooking Time: 0

Servings: 1

Ingredients :

• One handful of kale

• one banana, frozen

• Two cups of hemp seed milk

• One inch of ginger, finely minced

• Half cup of chopped strawberries, frozen

• 1 tablespoon of agave or your preferred sweetener

Directions:

1. Mix all the Ingredients in a blender and mix on high speed.

2. Allow it to blend evenly.

3. Pour into a pitcher with a few decorative straws and voila you are one happy camper.

4. Enjoy!

Nutrition:

Calories: 350

Fat: 4g

Carbohydrates: 52g

Protein: 16g

Orange Mixed Detox Smoothie

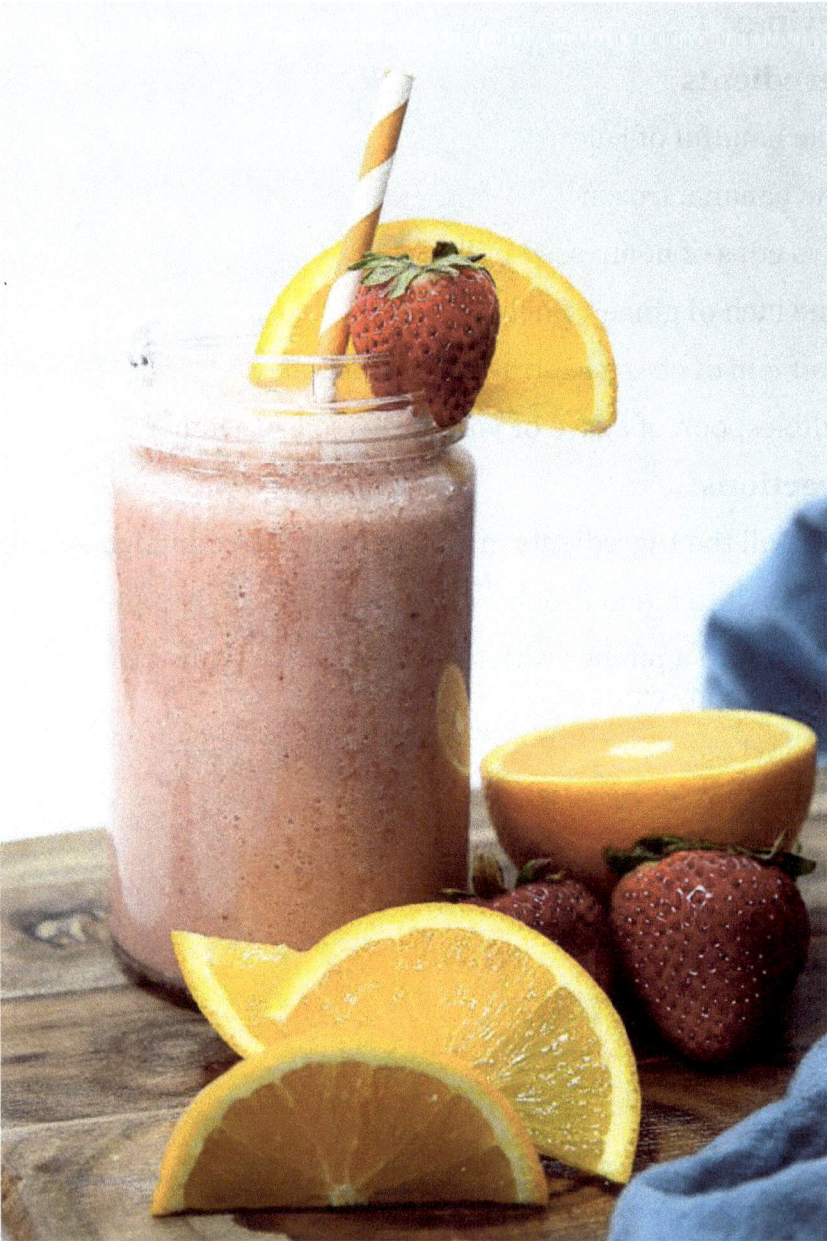

Preparation Time: 15 minutes

Cooking Time: 0

Servings: 1

Ingredients :

• One cup of vegies (Amaranth, Dandelion, Lettuce or Watercress)

• Half avocado

• One cup of tender-jelly coconut water

• One seville orange

• Juice of one key lime

• One tablespoon of bromide plus powder

Directions:

1. Peel and cut the Seville orange in chunks.

2. Mix all the Ingredients collectively in a high-speed blender until done.

Nutrition:

Calories: 71

Fat: 1g

Carbohydrates: 12g

Protein: 2g

Cucumber Toxin Flush Smoothie

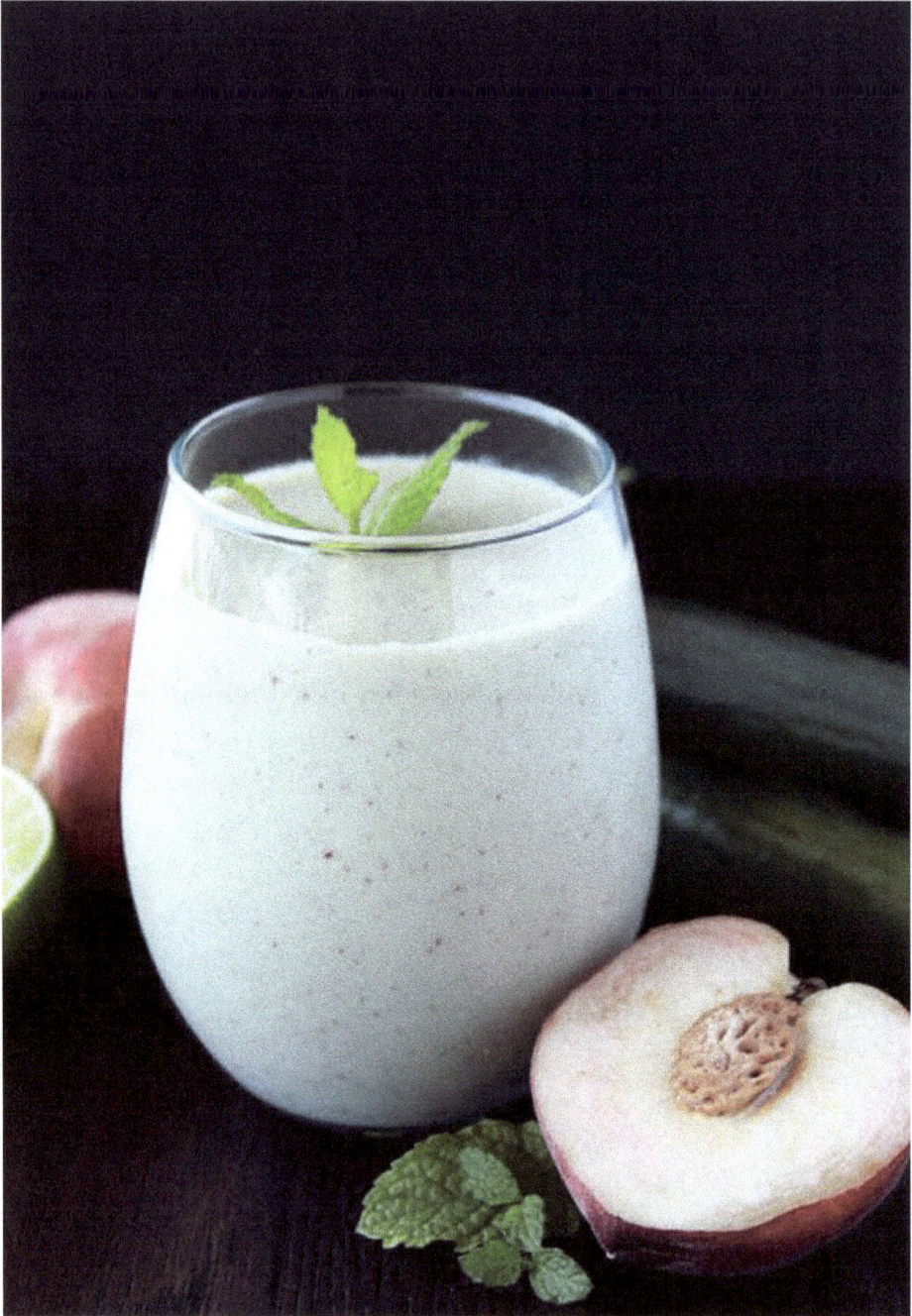

Preparation Time: 15 minutes

Cooking Time: 0

Servings: 1

Ingredients :

• 1 Cucumber

• 1 Key Lime

• 1 cup of watermelon (seeded), cubed

Directions:

1. Mix all the above Ingredients in a high-speed blender.

2. Considering that watermelon and cucumbers are largely water, you may not want to add any extra, however you can so if you want.

3. Juice the key lime and add into your smoothie.

4. Enjoy!

Nutrition:

Calories: 219

Fat: 4g

Carbohydrates: 48g

Protein: 5g

Apple Blueberry Smoothie

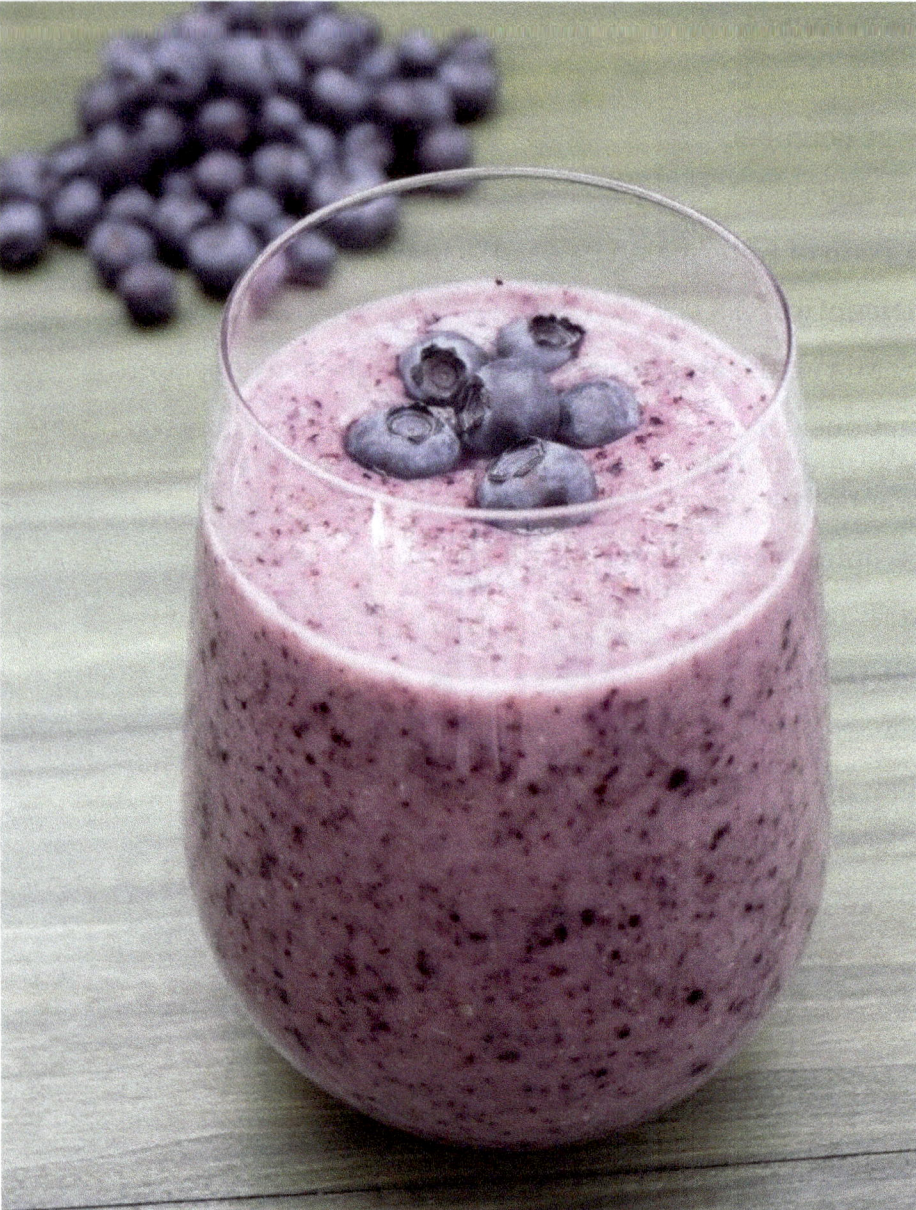

Preparation Time: 15 minutes

Cooking Time: 0

Servings: 1

Ingredients :

• Half apple

• One Date

• Half cup of blueberries

• Half cup of sparkling callaloo

• One tablespoon of hemp seeds

• One tablespoon of sesame seeds

• Two cups of sparkling soft-jelly coconut water

• Half of tablespoon of bromide plus powder

Directions:

1. Mix all of the Ingredients in a high-speed blender and enjoy!

Nutrition:

Calories: 167.4

Fat: 6.4g

Carbohydrates: 22.5g

Protein: 6.7g

Blueberry Smoothie

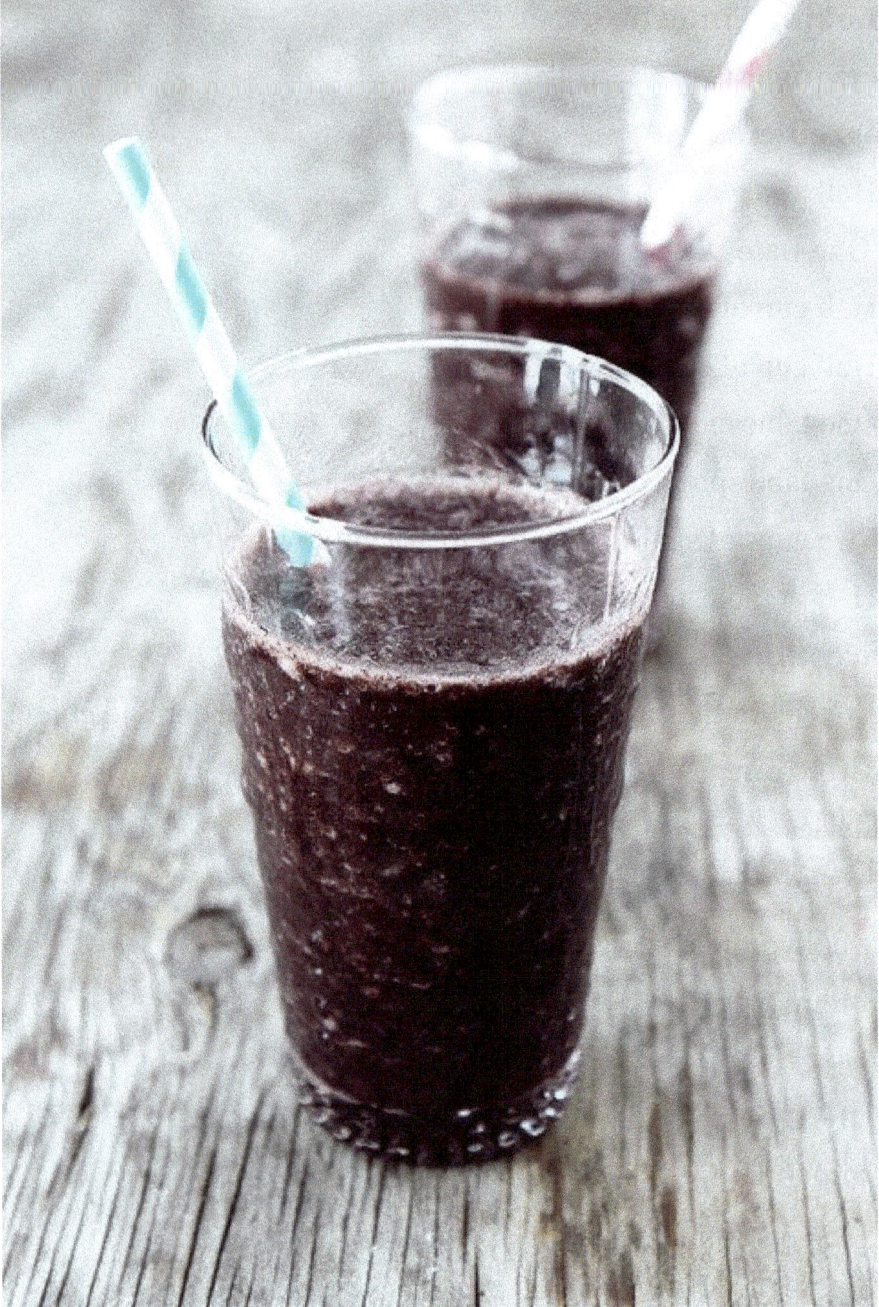

Preparation Time: 10 minutes

Cooking Time: 0 minutes

Servings: 2

Ingredients :

- 2 cups frozen blueberries
- 1 small banana
- 1½ cups unsweetened almond milk
- ¼ cup ice cubes

Directions:

1. Place all the Ingredients in a high-speed blender and pulse until creamy.

2. Pour the smoothie into two glasses and serve immediately.

Nutrition:

Calories 158

Total Fat 3.3 g

Saturated Fat 0.3 g

Cholesterol 0 mg

Sodium 137 mg

Total Carbs 34 g

Fiber 5.6 g

Sugar 20.6 g

Protein 2.4 g

Beet & Strawberry Smoothie

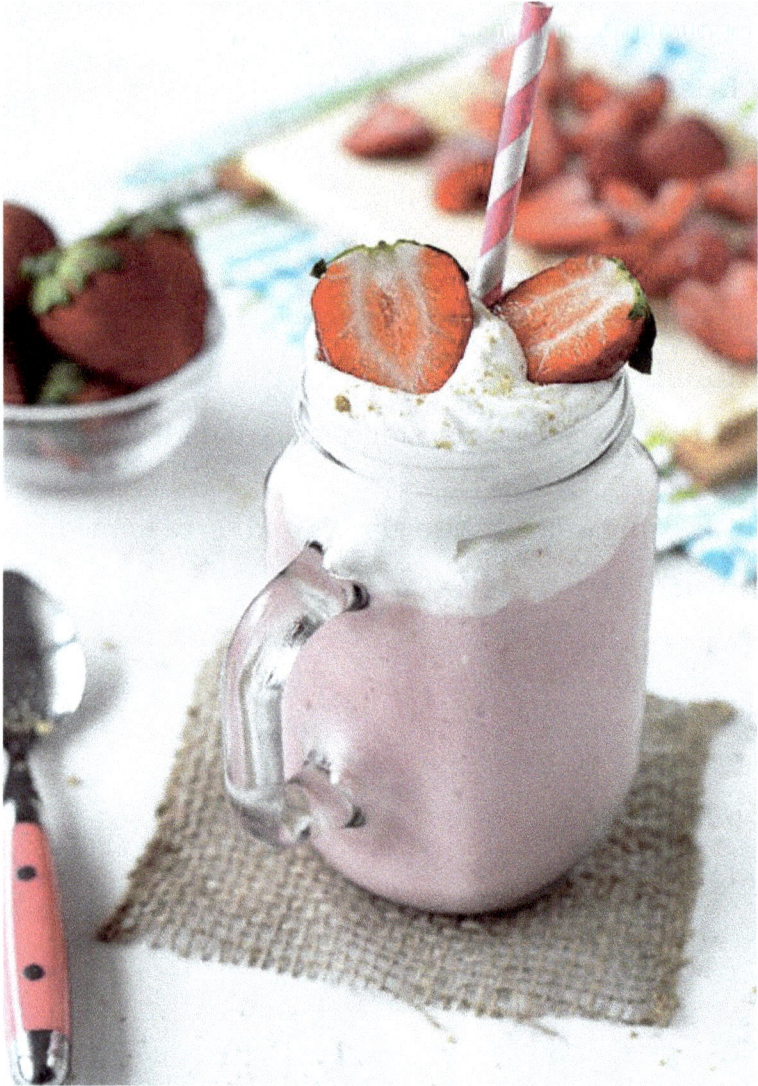

Preparation Time: 10 minutes

Cooking Time: 0 minutes

Servings: 2

Ingredients :

• 2 cups frozen strawberries, pitted and chopped

• **Servings:** cup roasted and frozen beet, chopped

• 1 teaspoon fresh ginger, peeled and grated

• 1 teaspoon fresh turmeric, peeled and grated

• ½ cup fresh orange juice

• 1 cup unsweetened almond milk

Directions:

1. Place all the Ingredients in a high-speed blender and pulse until creamy.

2. Pour the smoothie into two glasses and serve immediately.

Nutrition:

Calories 258

Total Fat 1.5 g

Saturated Fat 0.1 g

Cholesterol 0 mg

Sodium 134 mg

Total Carbs 26.7g

Fiber 4.9 g

Sugar 18.7 g

Protein 2.9 g

Kiwi Smoothie

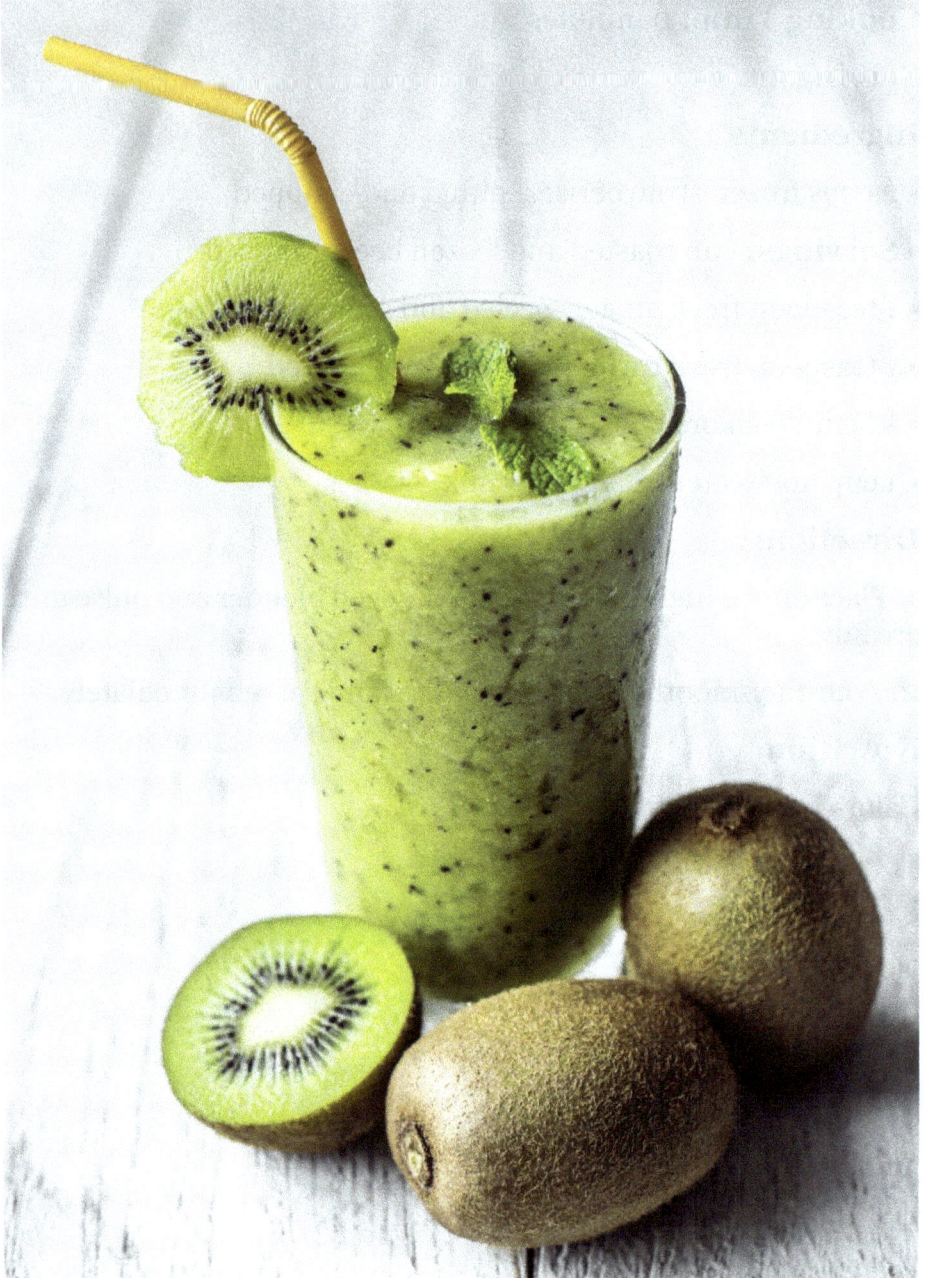

Preparation Time: 10 minutes

Cooking Time: 0 minutes

Servings: 2

Ingredients :

• 4 kiwis

• 2 small bananas, peeled

• 1½ cups unsweetened almond milk

• 1-2 drops liquid stevia

• ¼ cup ice cubes

Directions:

1. Place all the Ingredients in a high-speed blender and pulse until creamy.

2. Pour the smoothie into two glasses and serve immediately.

Nutrition:

Calories 228

Total Fat 3.8 g

Saturated Fat 0.4 g

Cholesterol 0 mg

Sodium 141 mg

Total Carbs 50.7 g

Fiber 8.4 g

Sugar 28.1 g

Protein 3.8 g

Pineapple & Carrot Smoothie

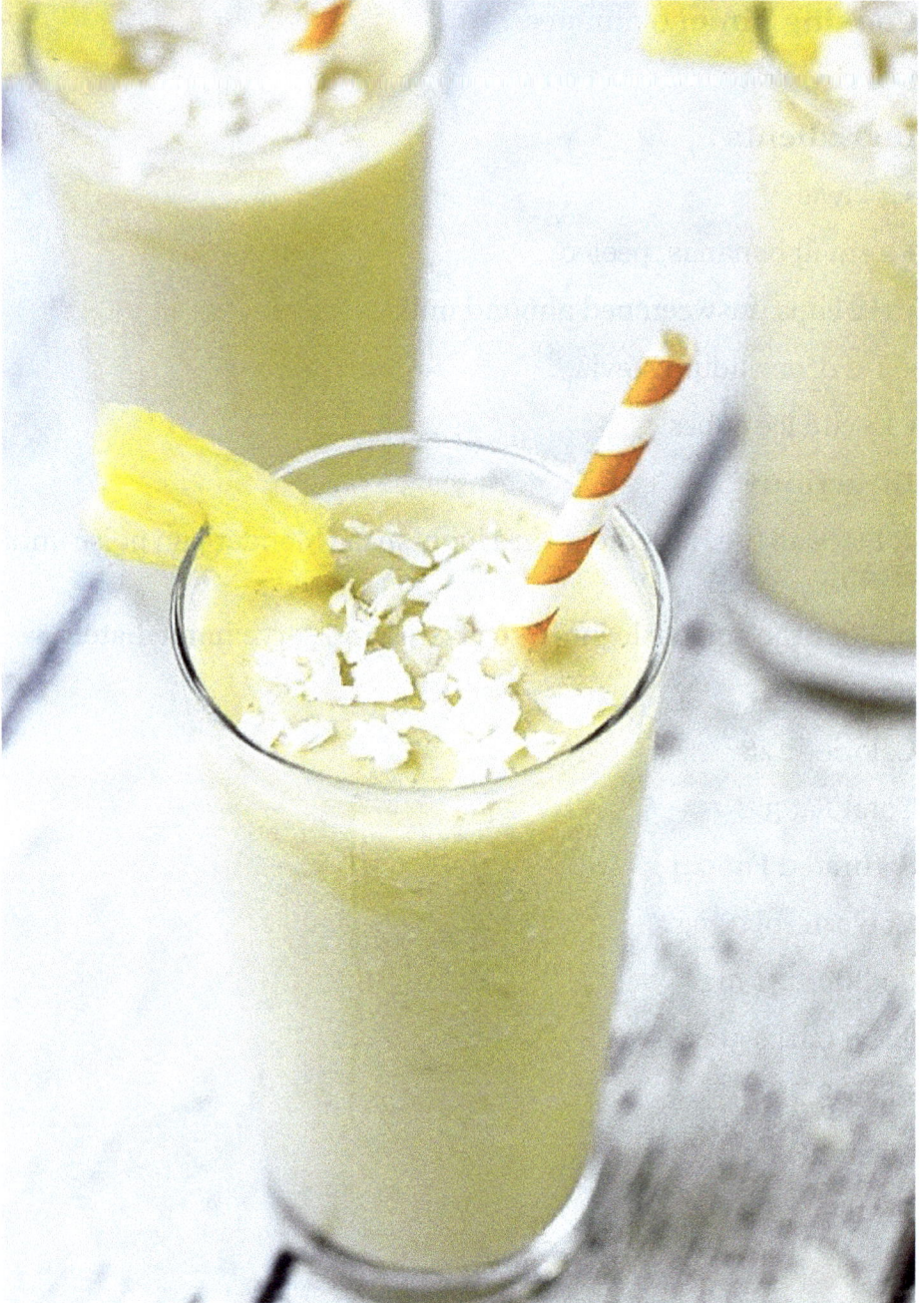

Preparation Time: 10 minutes

Cooking Time: 0 minutes

Servings: 2

Ingredients :

- 1 cup frozen pineapple
- 1 large ripe banana, peeled and sliced
- ½ tablespoon fresh ginger, peeled and chopped
- ¼ teaspoon ground turmeric
- 1 cup unsweetened almond milk
- ½ cup fresh carrot juice
- 1 tablespoon fresh lemon juice

Directions:

1. Place all the Ingredients in a high-speed blender and pulse until creamy.

2. Pour the smoothie into two glasses and serve immediately.

Nutrition:

Calories 132

Total Fat 2.2 g

Saturated Fat 0.3 g

Cholesterol 0 mg

Sodium 113 mg

Total Carbs 629.3 g

Fiber 4.1 g

Sugar 16.9 g

Protein 2 g

Oats & Orange Smoothie

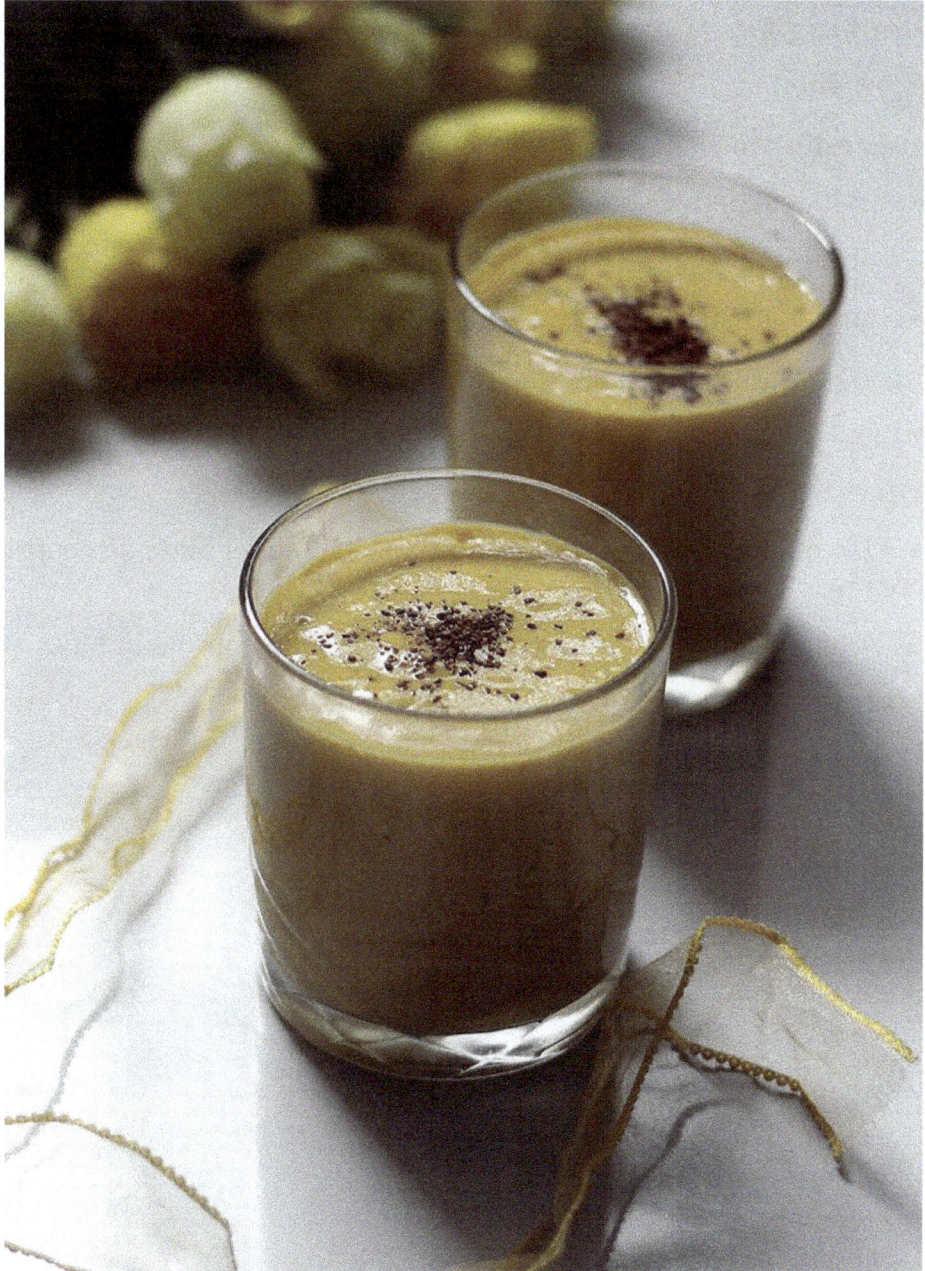

Preparation Time: 10 minutes

Cooking Time: 0 minutes

Servings: 4

Ingredients :

• Servings: cup rolled oats

• 2 oranges, peeled, seeded, and sectioned

• 2 large bananas, peeled and sliced

• 2 cups unsweetened almond milk

• 1 cup ice cubes, crushed

Directions:

1. Place all the Ingredients in a high-speed blender and pulse until creamy.

2. Pour the smoothie into four glasses and serve immediately.

Nutrition:

Calories 175

Total Fat 3 g

Saturated Fat 0.4 g

Cholesterol 0 mg

Sodium 93 mg

Total Carbs 36.6 g

Fiber 5.9 g

Sugar 17.1 g

Protein 3.9 g

Pumpkin Creamed Smoothie

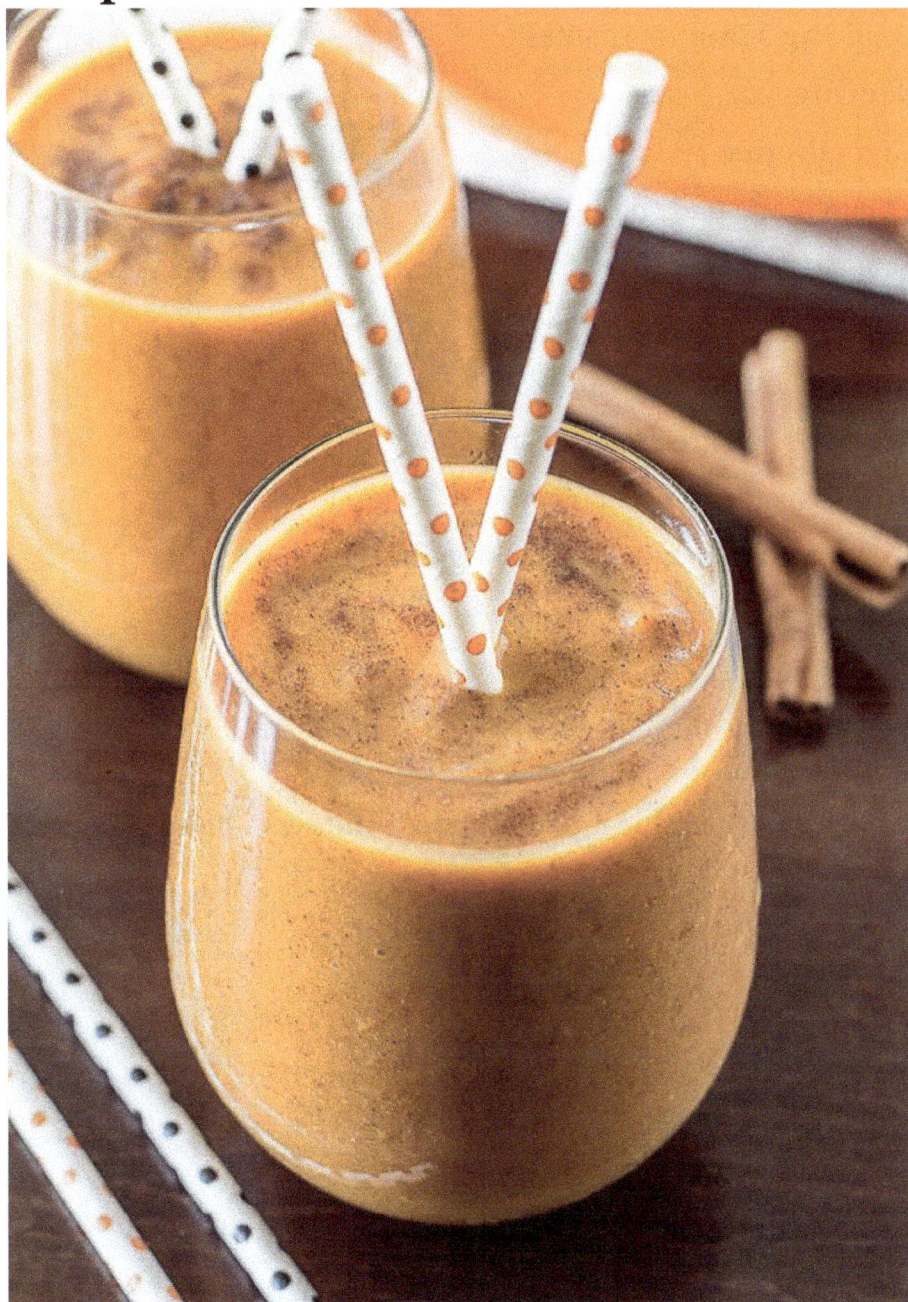

Preparation Time: 10 minutes

Cooking Time: 0 minutes

Servings: 2

Ingredients :

- 1 cup homemade pumpkin puree
- 1 medium banana, peeled and sliced
- 1 tablespoon maple syrup
- 1 teaspoon ground flaxseeds
- ½ teaspoon ground cinnamon
- ¼ teaspoon ground ginger
- 1½ cups unsweetened almond milk
- ¼ cup ice cubes

Directions:

1. Place all the Ingredients in a high-speed blender and pulse until creamy.

2. Pour the smoothie into two glasses and serve immediately.

Nutrition:

Calories 159

Total Fat 3.6 g

Saturated Fat 0.5 g

Cholesterol 0 mg

Sodium 143 mg

Total Carbs 32.6 g

Fiber 6.5 g

Sugar 17.3 g

Protein 3 g

Red Veggie & Fruit Smoothie

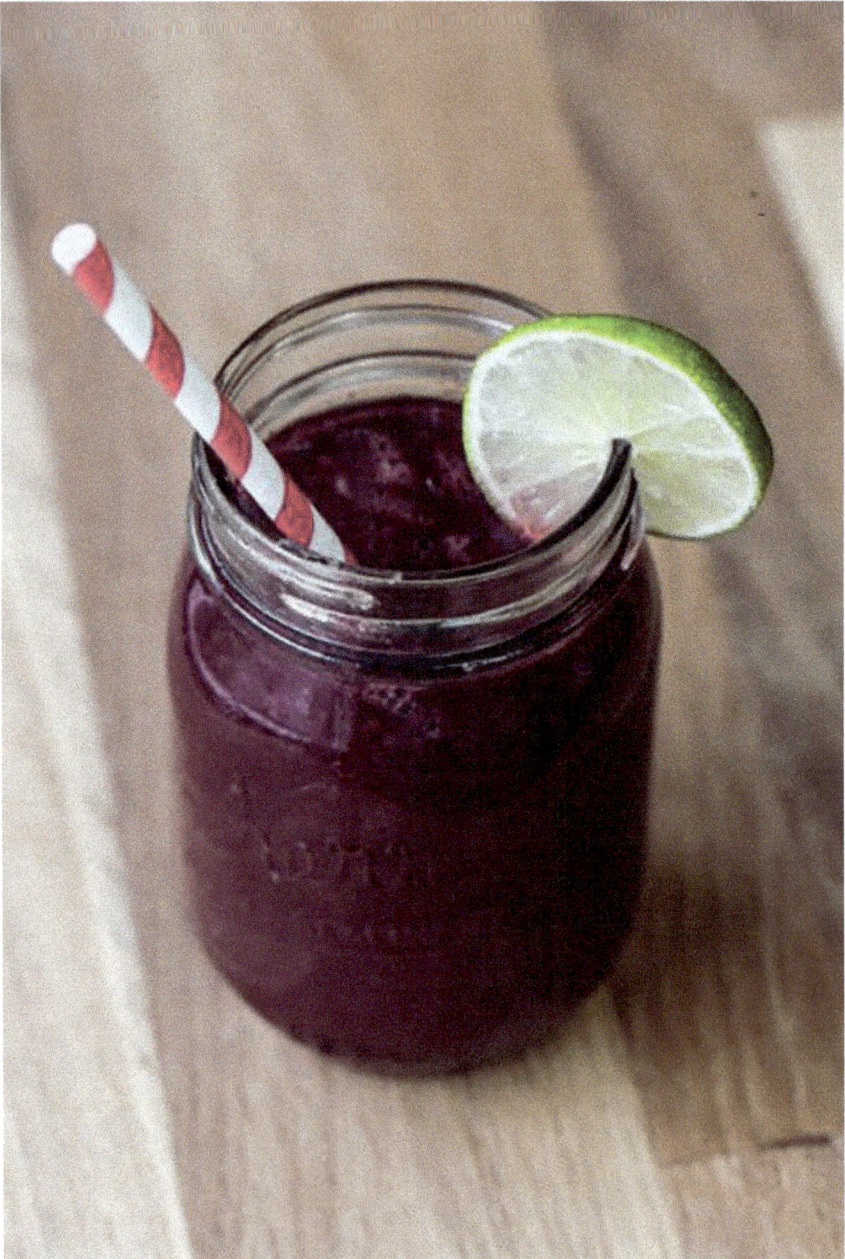

Preparation Time: 10 minutes

Cooking Time: 0 minutes

Servings: 2

Ingredients :

- ½ cup fresh raspberries
- ½ cup fresh strawberries
- ½ red bell pepper, seeded and chopped
- ½ cup red cabbage, chopped
- 1 small tomato
- 1 cup water
- ½ cup ice cubes

Directions:

1. Place all the Ingredients in a high-speed blender and pulse until creamy.

2. Pour the smoothie into two glasses and serve immediately.

Nutrition:

Calories 39

Cholesterol 0 mg

Saturated Fat 0 g

Sodium 10 mg

Total Carbs 8.9 g

Fiber 3.5 g

Sugar 4.8 g

Protein 1.3 g

Total Fat 0.4 g

Kale Smoothie

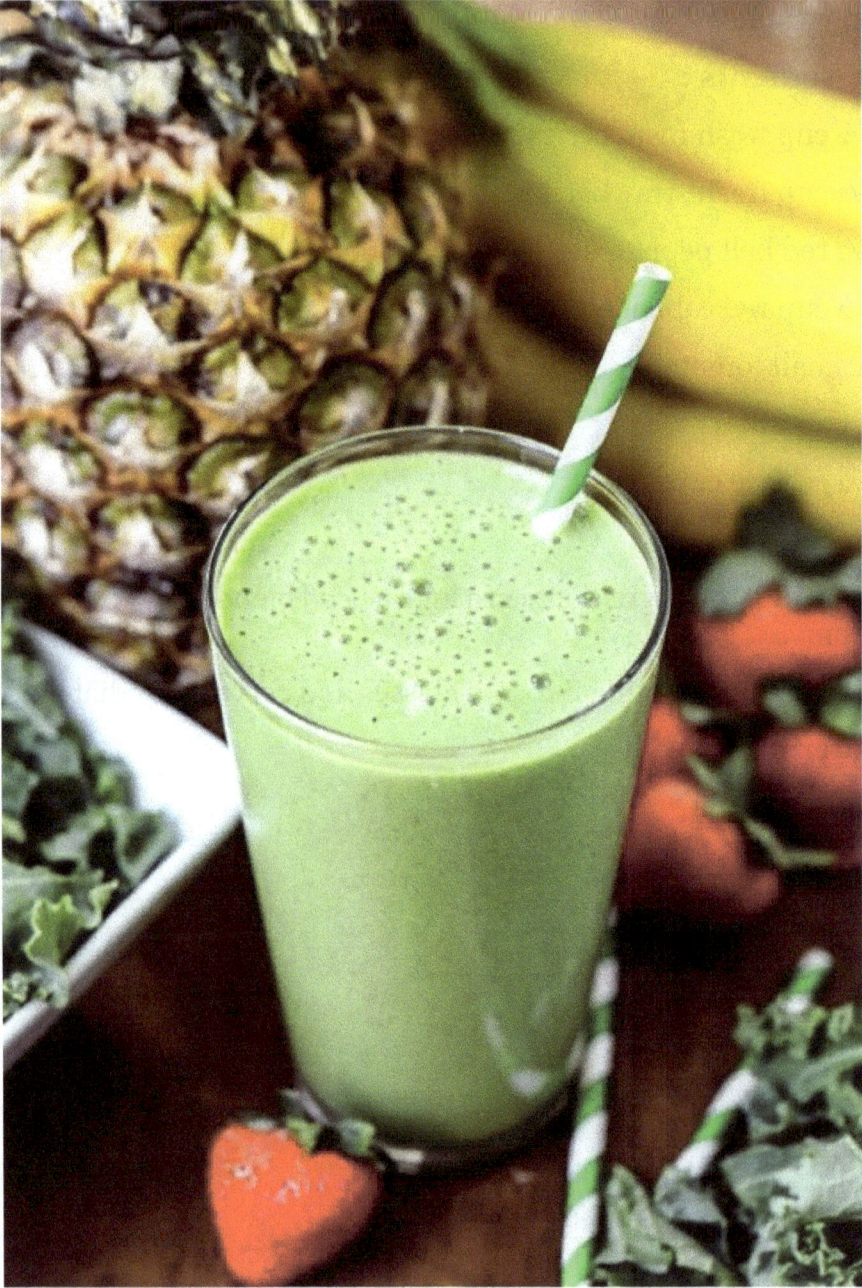

Preparation Time: 10 minutes

Cooking Time: 0 minutes

Servings: 2

Ingredients :

- 3 stalks fresh kale, trimmed and chopped
- 1-2 celery stalks, chopped
- ½ avocado, peeled, pitted, and chopped
- ½-inch piece ginger root, chopped
- ½-inch piece turmeric root, chopped
- 2 cups coconut milk

Directions:

1. Place all the Ingredients in a high-speed blender and pulse until creamy.

2. Pour the smoothie into two glasses and serve immediately.

Nutrition:

Calories 248

Total Fat 22.8 g

Saturated Fat 12 g

Cholesterol 0 mg

Sodium 59 mg

Total Carbs 11.3 g

Fiber 4.2 g

Sugar 0.5 g

Protein 3.5 g

Green Tofu Smoothie

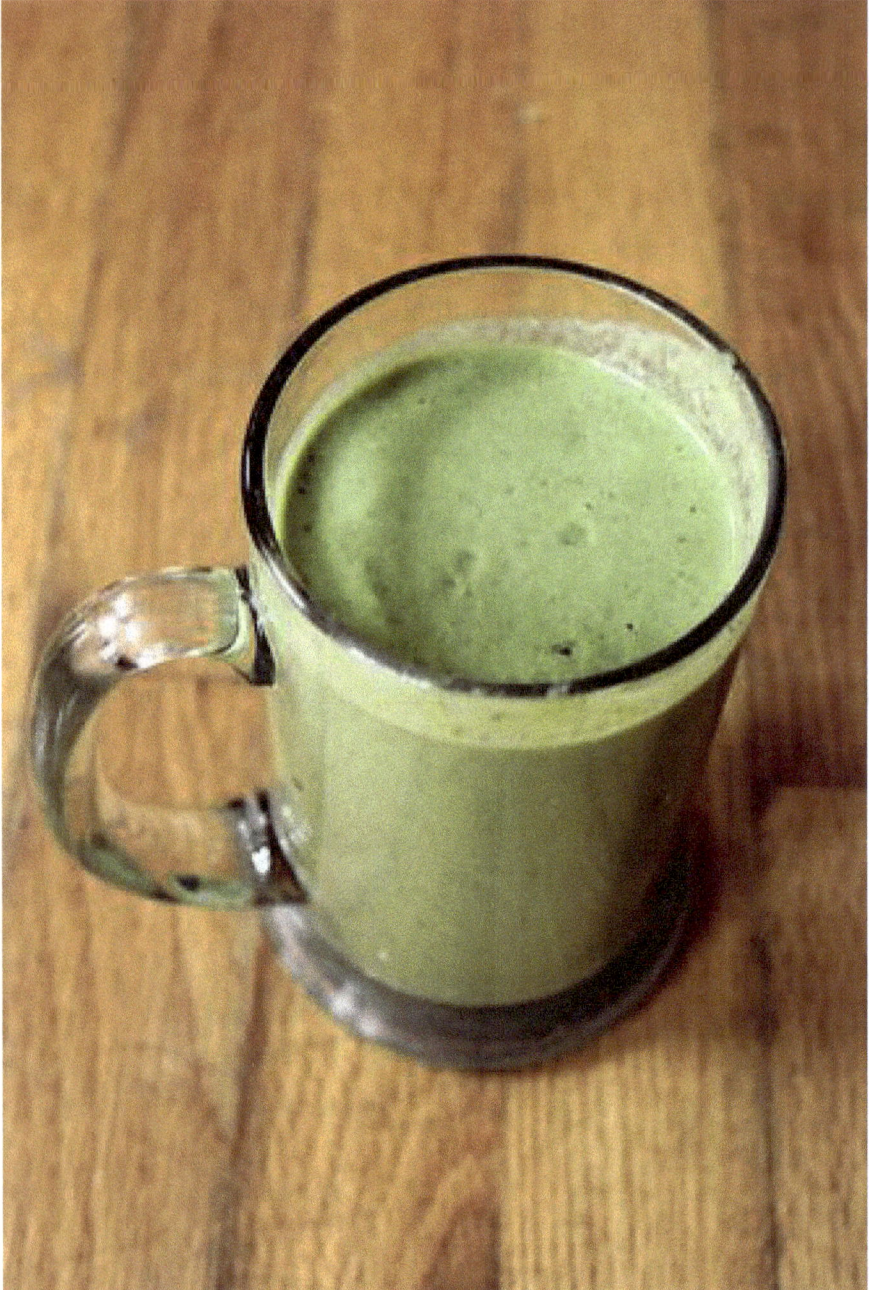

Preparation Time: 10 minutes

Cooking Time: 0 minutes

Servings: 2

Ingredients :

• 1½ cups cucumber, peeled and chopped roughly

• 3 cups fresh baby spinach

• 2 cups frozen broccoli

• ½ cup silken tofu, drained and pressed

• 1 tablespoon fresh lime juice

• 4-5 drops liquid stevia

• 1 cup unsweetened almond milk

• ½ cup ice, crushed

Directions:

1. Place all the Ingredients in a high-speed blender and pulse until creamy.

2. Pour the smoothie into two glasses and serve immediately.

Nutrition:

Calories 118

Total Fat 15 g

Saturated Fat 0.8 g

Cholesterol 0 mg

Sodium 165 mg

Total Carbs 12.6 g

Fiber 4.8 g

Sugar 3.4 g

Protein 10 g

Grape & Swiss Chard Smoothie

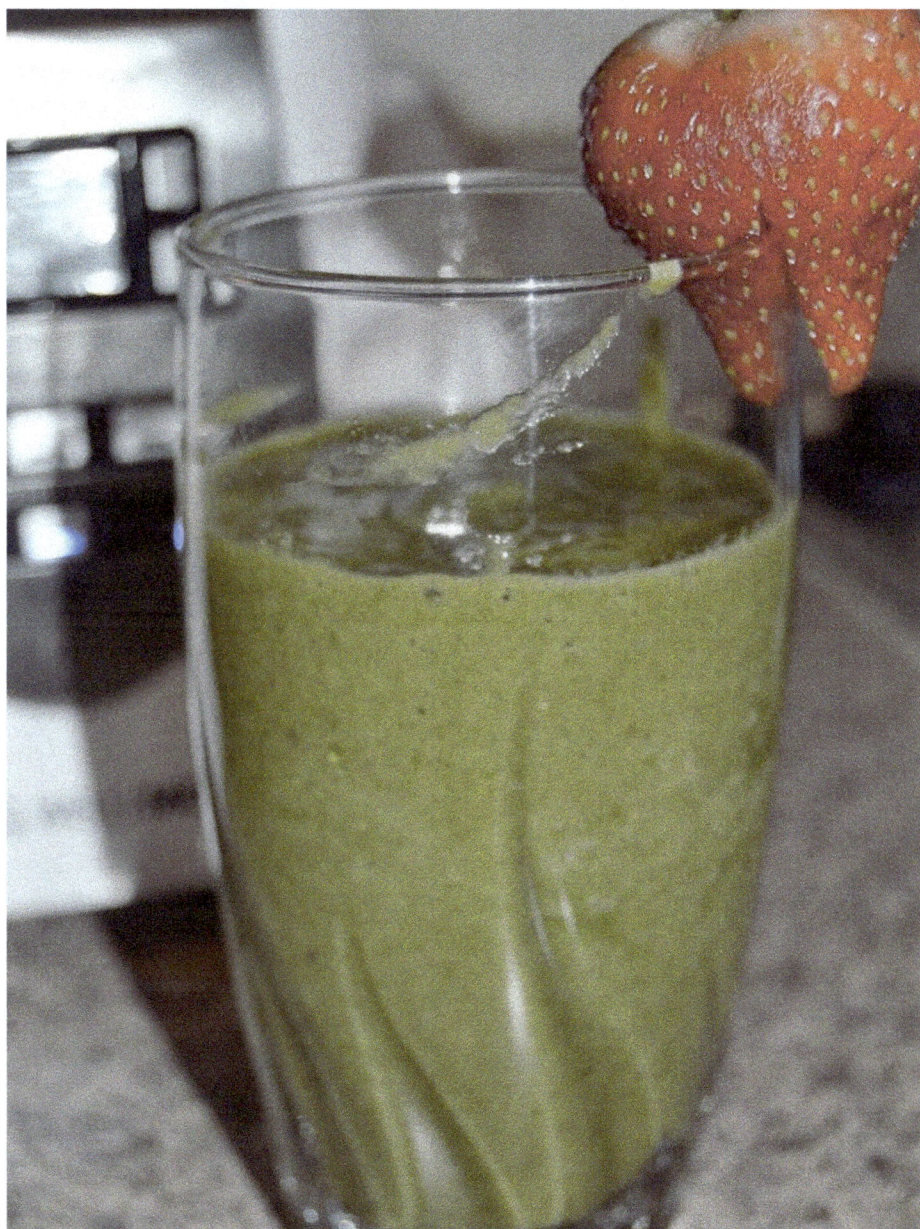

Preparation Time: 10 minutes

Cooking Time: 0 minutes

Servings: 2

Ingredients :

- 2 cups seedless green grapes
- 2 cups fresh Swiss chard, trimmed and chopped
- 2 tablespoons maple syrup
- 1 teaspoon fresh lemon juice
- 1½ cups water
- 4 ice cubes

Directions:

1. Place all the Ingredients in a high-speed blender and pulse until creamy.

2. Pour the smoothie into two glasses and serve immediately.

Nutrition:

Calories 176

Total Fat 0.2 g

Saturated Fat 0 g

Cholesterol 0 mg

Sodium 83 mg

Total Carbs 44.9 g

Fiber 1.7 g

Sugar 37.9 g

Protein 0.7 g

Matcha Creamed Smoothie

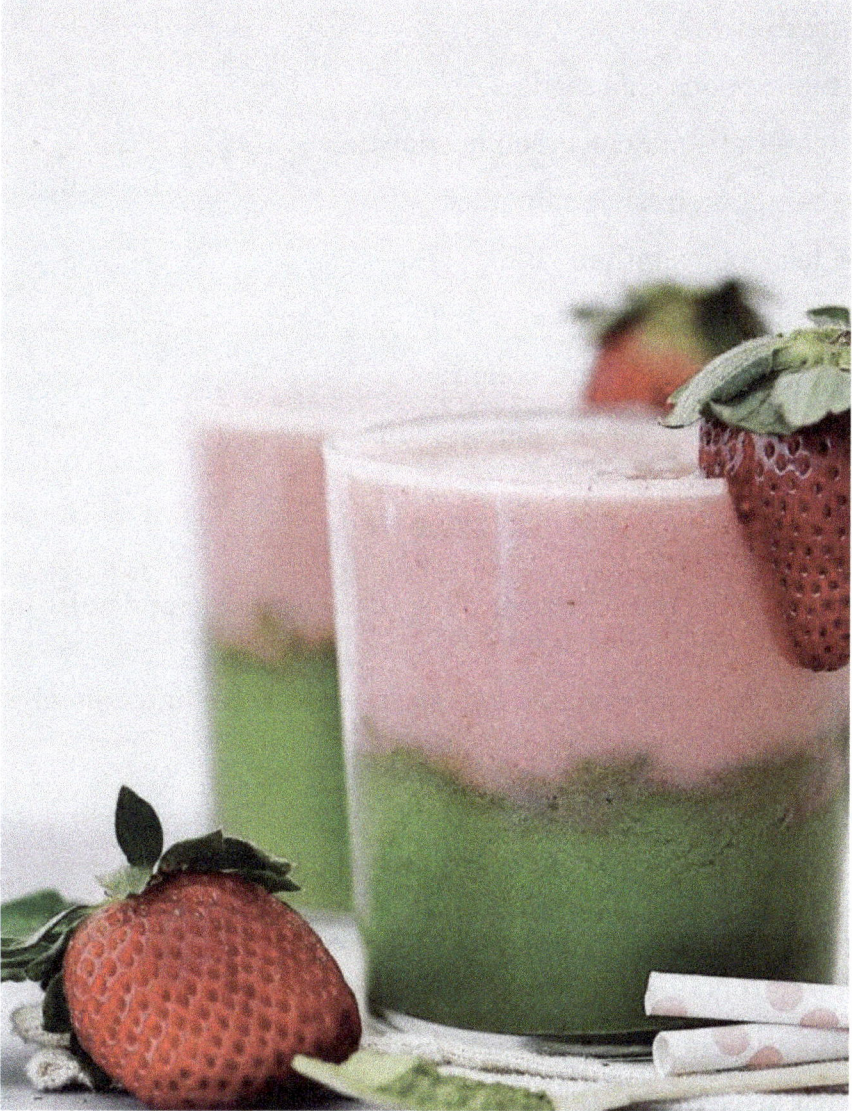

Preparation Time: 10 minutes

Cooking Time: 0 minutes

Servings: 2

Ingredients :

- 2 tablespoons chia seeds
- 2 teaspoons matcha green tea powder
- ½ teaspoon fresh lemon juice
- ½ teaspoon xanthan gum
- 8-10 drops liquid stevia
- 4 tablespoons coconut cream
- 1½ cups unsweetened almond milk
- ¼ cup ice cubes

Directions:

1. Place all the Ingredients in a high-speed blender and pulse until creamy.

2. Pour the smoothie into two glasses and serve immediately.

Nutrition:

Calories 132

Total Fat 12.3 g

Saturated Fat 6.8 g

Cholesterol 0 mg

Sodium 15 mg

Total Carbs 7 g

Fiber 4.8 g

Sugar 1 g

Protein 3 g

Banana Smoothie

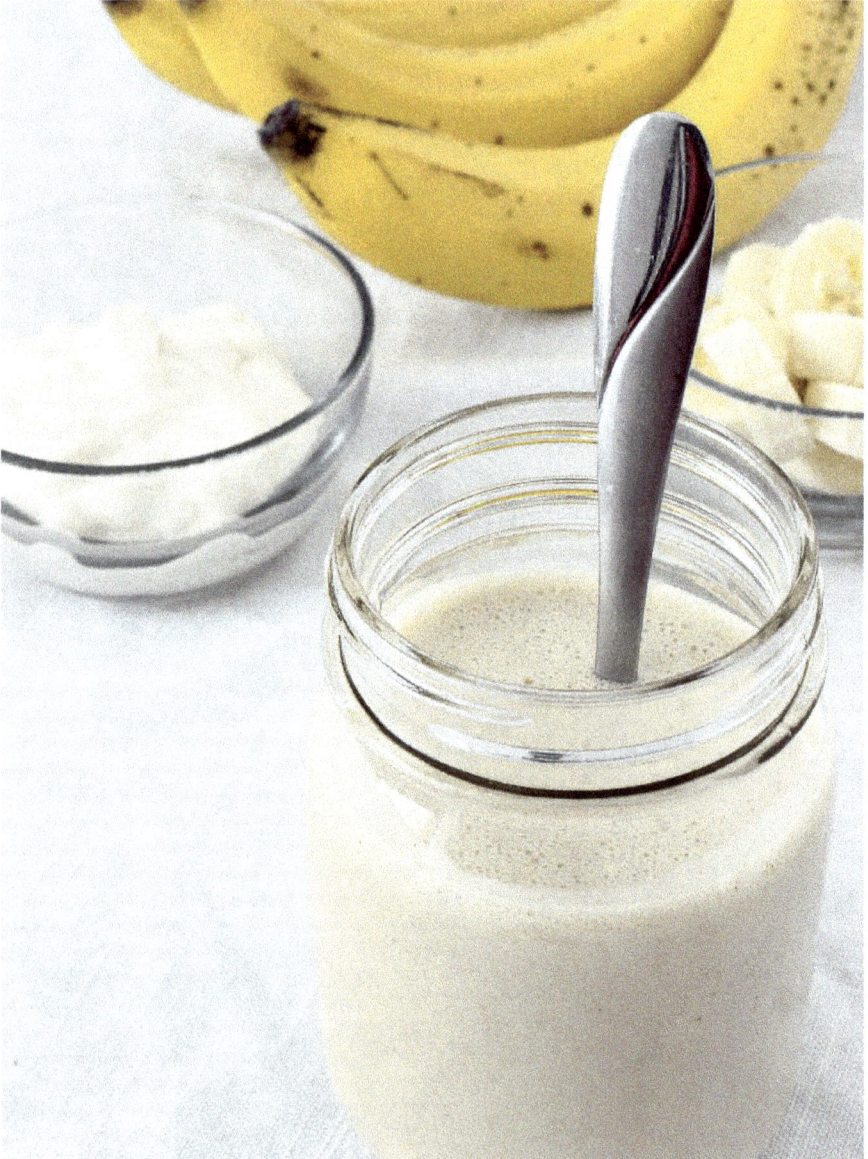

Preparation Time: 10 minutes

Cooking Time: 0 minutes

Servings: 2

Ingredients :

- 2 cups chilled unsweetened almond milk
- 1 large frozen banana, peeled and sliced
- 1 tablespoon almonds, chopped
- 1 teaspoon organic vanilla extract

Directions:

1. Place all the Ingredients in a high-speed blender and pulse until creamy.

2. Pour the smoothie into two glasses and serve immediately.

Nutrition:

Calories 124

Total Fat 5.2 g

Saturated Fat 0.5 g

Cholesterol 0 mg

Sodium 181 mg

Total Carbs 18.4 g

Fiber 3.1 g

Sugar 8.7 g

Protein 2.4 g

Strawberry Creamed Smoothie

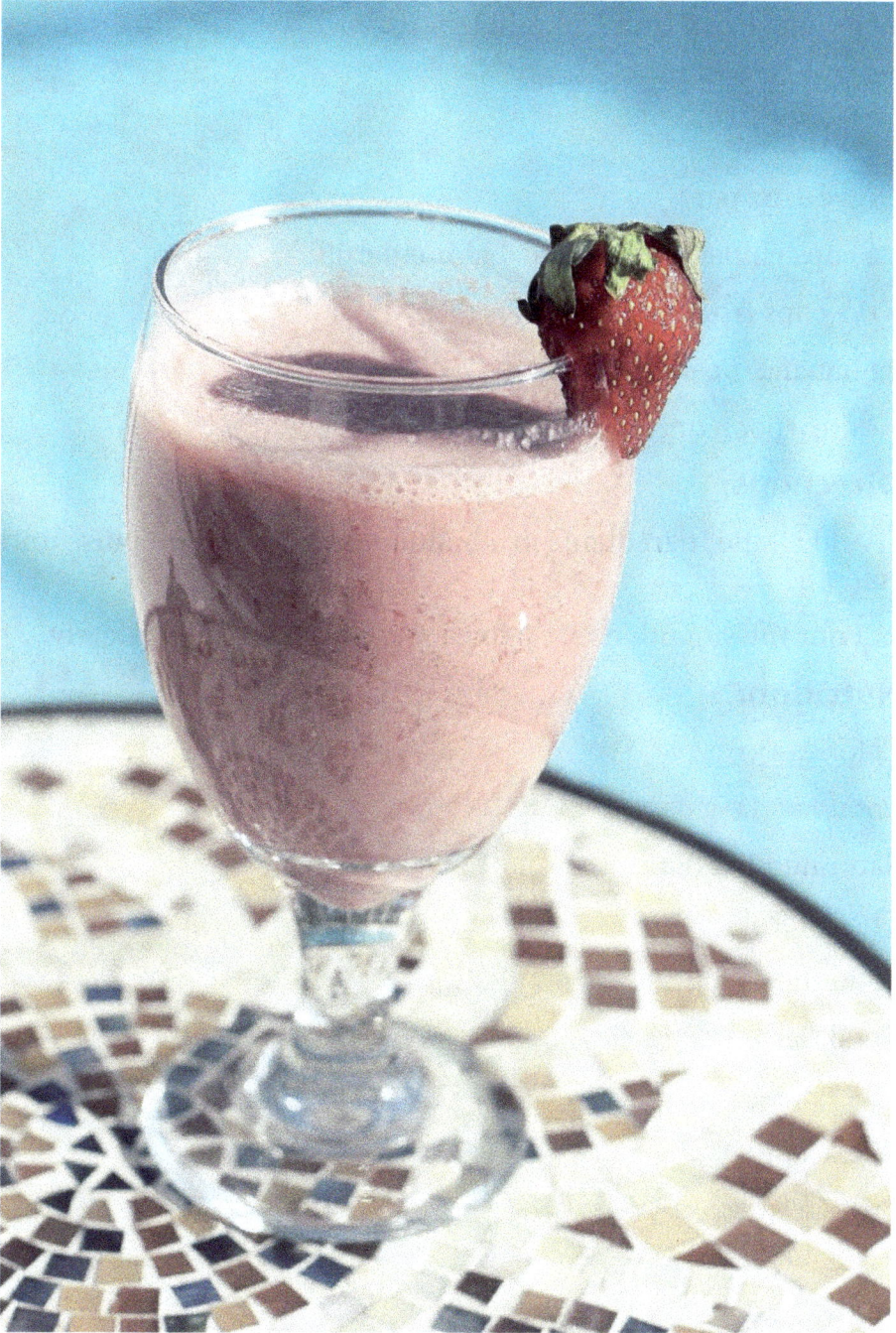

Preparation Time: 10 minutes

Cooking Time: 0 minutes

Servings: 2

Ingredients :

- 2 cups chilled unsweetened almond milk
- 1½ cups frozen strawberries
- 1 banana, peeled and sliced
- ¼ teaspoon organic vanilla extract

Directions:

1. Add all the Ingredients in a high-speed blender and pulse until smooth.

2. Pour the smoothie into two glasses and serve immediately.

Nutrition:

Calories 131

Total Fat 3.7 g

Saturated Fat 0.4 g

Cholesterol 0 mg

Sodium 181 mg

Total Carbs 25.3 g

Fiber 4.8 g

Sugar 14 g

Protein 1.6 g

Raspberry & Tofu Smoothie

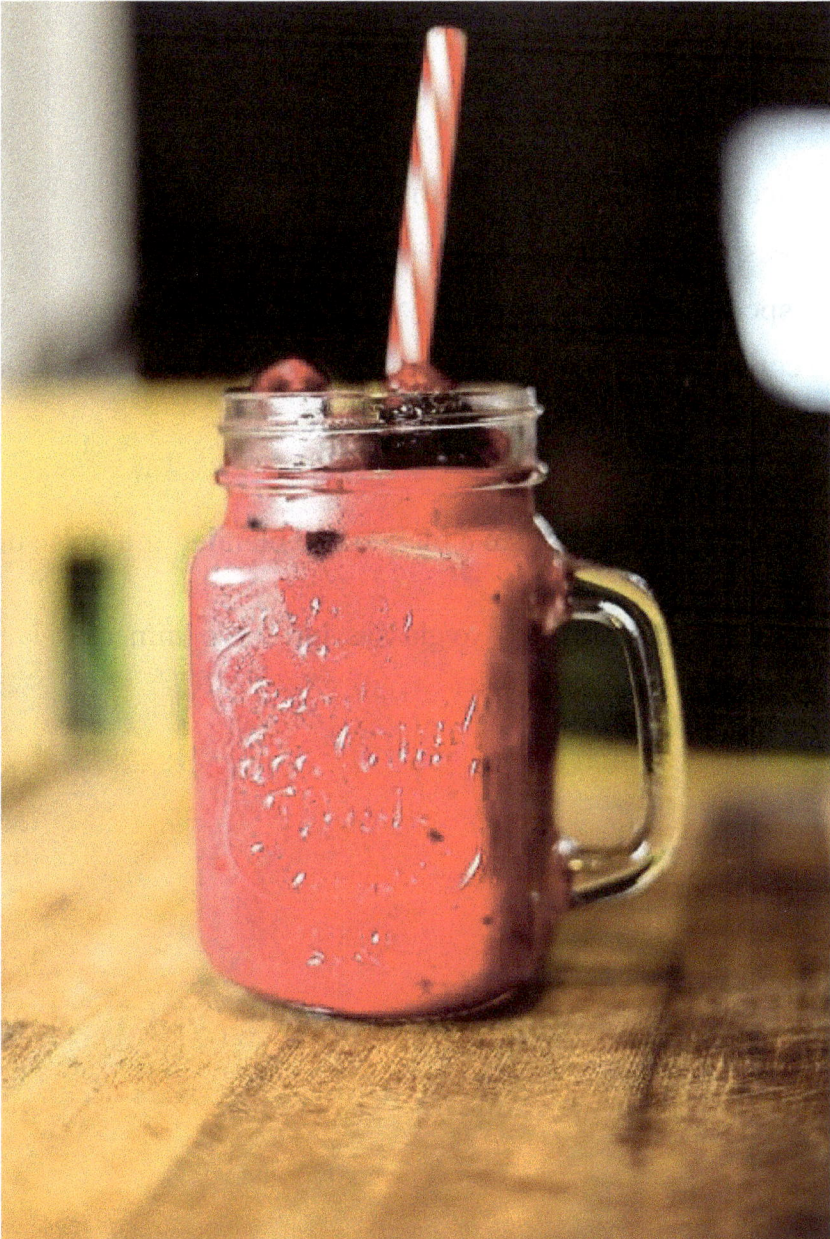

Preparation Time: 15 minutes

Cooking Time: 0 minutes

Servings: 2

Ingredients :

- 1½ cups fresh raspberries
- 6 ounces firm silken tofu, drained
- 1/8 teaspoon coconut extract
- 1 teaspoon powdered stevia
- 1½ cups unsweetened almond milk
- ¼ cup ice cubes, crushed

Directions:

1. Add all the Ingredients in a high-speed blender and pulse until smooth.

2. Pour the smoothie into two glasses and serve immediately.

Nutrition:

Calories 131

Total Fat 5.5 g

Saturated Fat 0.6 g

Cholesterol 0 mg

Sodium 167 mg

Total Carbs 14.6 g

Fiber 6.8 g

Sugar 5.2 g

Protein 7.7 g

Mango Smoothie

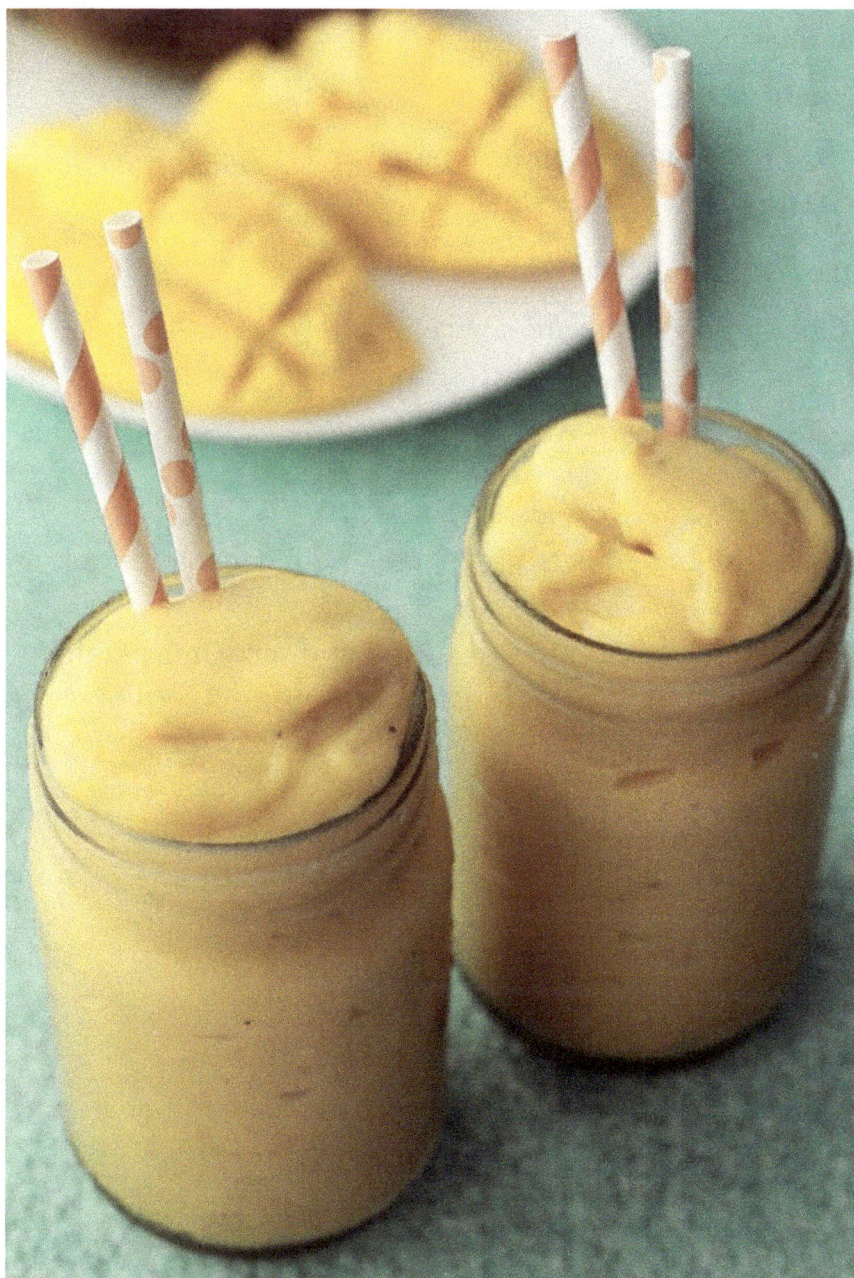

Preparation Time: 10 minutes

Cooking Time: 0 minutes

Servings. 2

Ingredients :

• 2 cups frozen mango, peeled, pitted and chopped

• ¼ cup almond butter

• Pinch of ground turmeric

• 2 tablespoons fresh lemon juice

• 1¼ cups unsweetened almond milk

• ¼ cup ice cubes

Directions:

1. Add all the Ingredients in a high-speed blender and pulse until smooth.

2. Pour the smoothie into two glasses and serve immediately.

Nutrition:

Calories 140

Total Fat 4.1 g

Saturated Fat 0.6 g

Cholesterol 0 mg

Sodium 118 mg

Total Carbs 26.8 g

Fiber 3.6 g

Sugar 23 g

Protein 2.5 g

Pineapple Smoothie

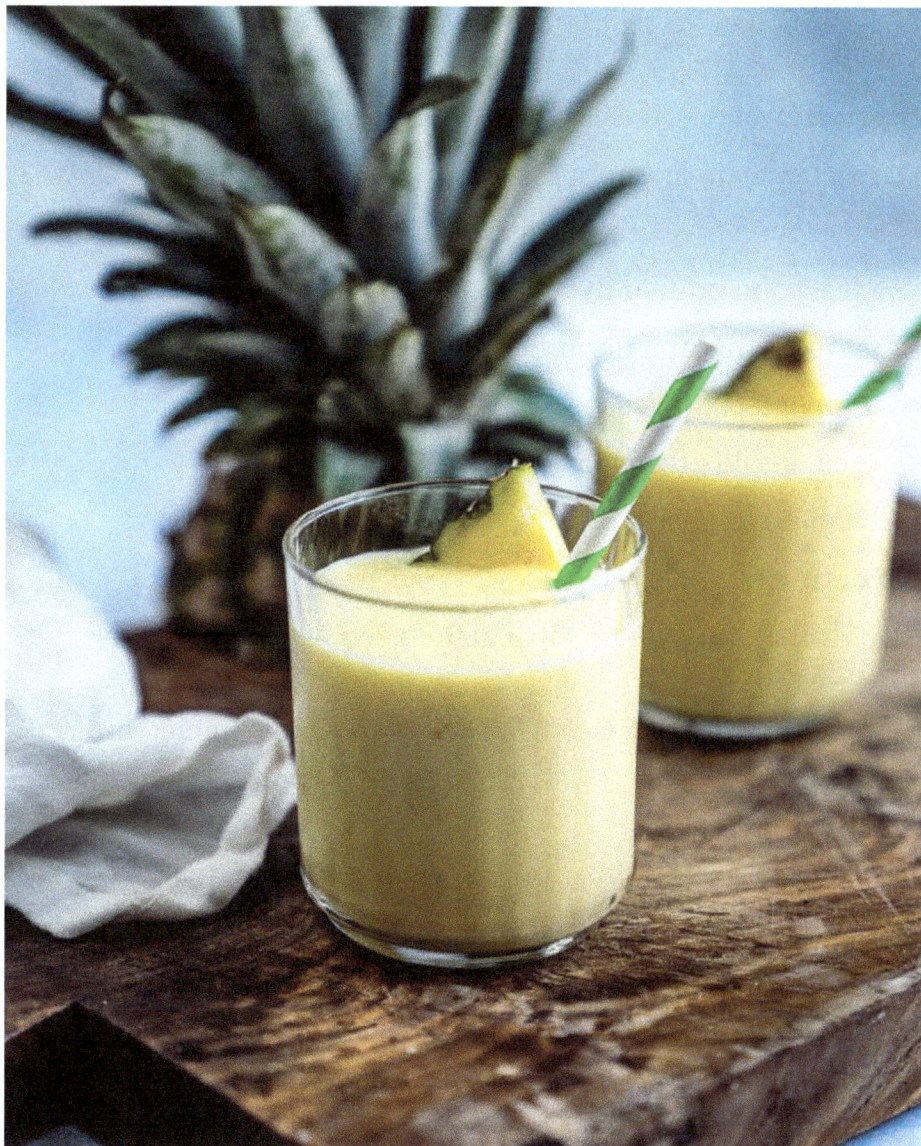

Preparation Time: 10 minutes

Cooking Time: 0 minutes

Servings: 2

Ingredients :

• 2 cups pineapple, chopped

• ½ teaspoon fresh ginger, peeled and chopped

• ½ teaspoon ground turmeric

• 1 teaspoon natural immune support supplement *

• 1 teaspoon chia seeds

• 1½ cups cold green tea

• ½ cup ice, crushed

Directions:

1. Add all the Ingredients in a high-speed blender and pulse until smooth.

2. Pour the smoothie into two glasses and serve immediately.

Nutrition:

Calories 152

Total Fat 1 g

Saturated Fat 0 g

Cholesterol 0 mg

Sodium 9 mg

Total Carbs 30 g

Fiber 3.5 g

Sugar 29.8 g

Protein 1.5 g

Kale & Pineapple Smoothie

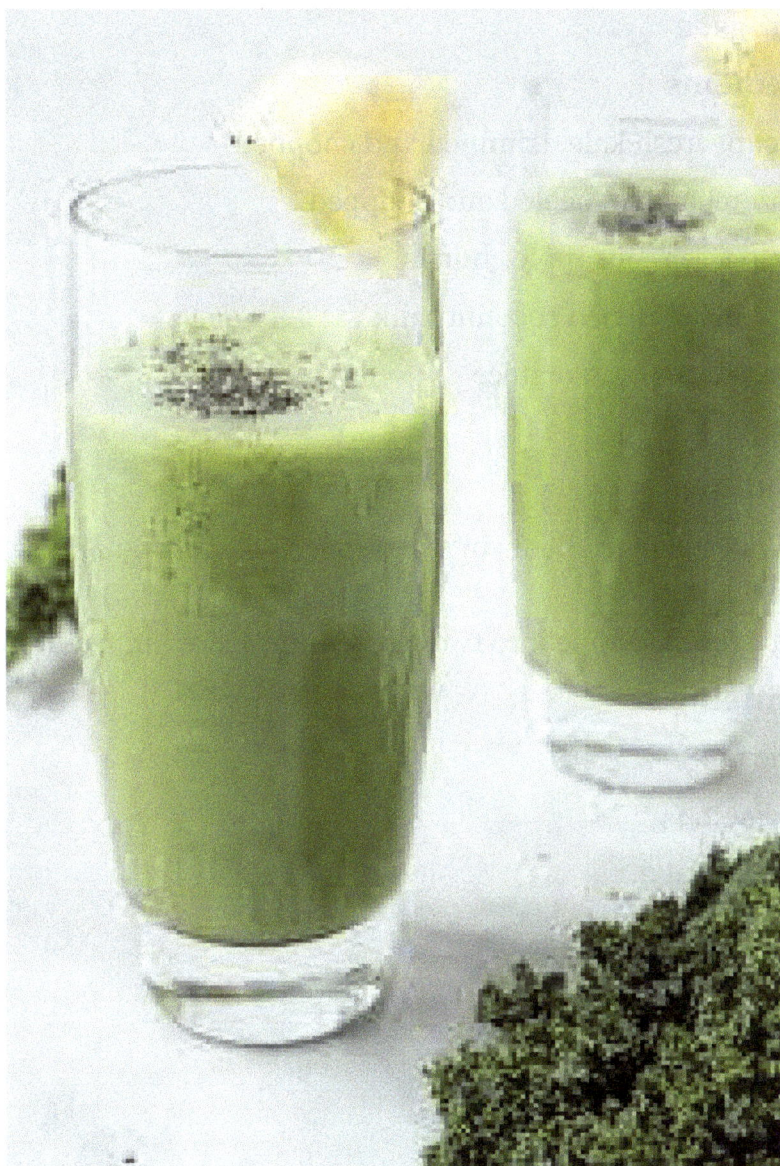

Preparation Time: 15 minutes

Cooking Time: 0 minutes

Servings: 2

Ingredients :

- 1½ cups fresh kale, trimmed and chopped
- 1 frozen banana, peeled and chopped
- ½ cup fresh pineapple chunks
- 1 cup unsweetened coconut milk
- ½ cup fresh orange juice
- ½ cup ice

Directions:

1. Add all the Ingredients in a high-speed blender and pulse until smooth.

2. Pour the smoothie into two glasses and serve immediately.

Nutrition:

Calories 148

Total Fat 2.4 g

Saturated Fat 2.1 g

Cholesterol 0 mg

Sodium 23 mg

Total Carbs 31.6 g

Fiber 3.5 g

Sugar 16.5 g

Protein 2.8 g

Green Veggies Smoothie

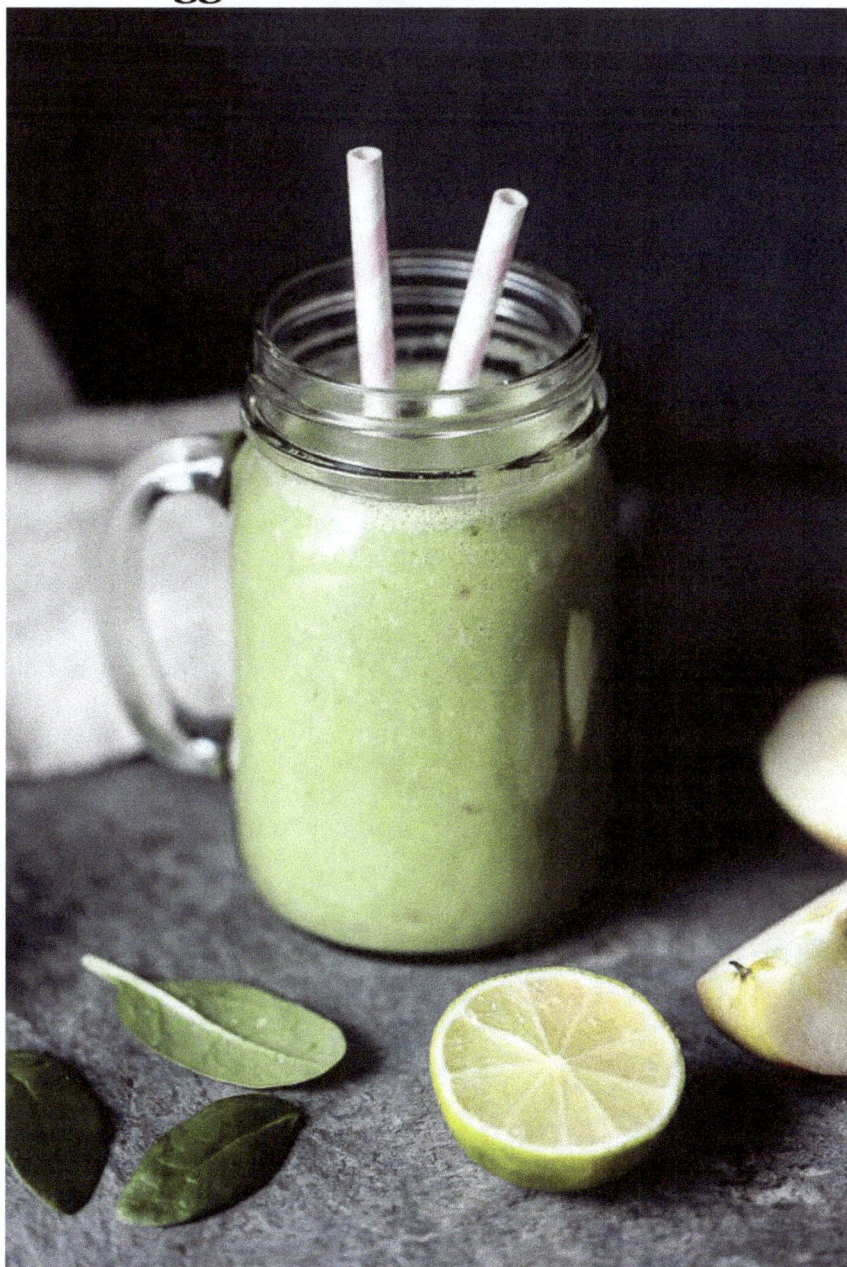

Preparation Time: 15 minutes

Cooking Time: 0 minutes

Servings: 2

Ingredients :

- 1 medium avocado, peeled, pitted, and chopped
- 1 large cucumber, peeled and chopped
- 2 fresh tomatoes, chopped
- 1 small green bell pepper, seeded and chopped
- 1 cup fresh spinach, torn
- 2 tablespoons fresh lime juice
- 2 tablespoons homemade vegetable broth
- 1 cup alkaline water

Directions:

1. Add all the Ingredients in a high-speed blender and pulse until smooth.

2. Pour the smoothie into glasses and serve immediately.

Nutrition:

Calories 275

Total Fat 20.3 g

Saturated Fat 4.2 g

Cholesterol 0 mg

Sodium 76 mg

Total Carbs 24.1 g

Fiber 10.1 g

Sugar 9.3 g

Protein 5.3 g

Avocado & Spinach Smoothie

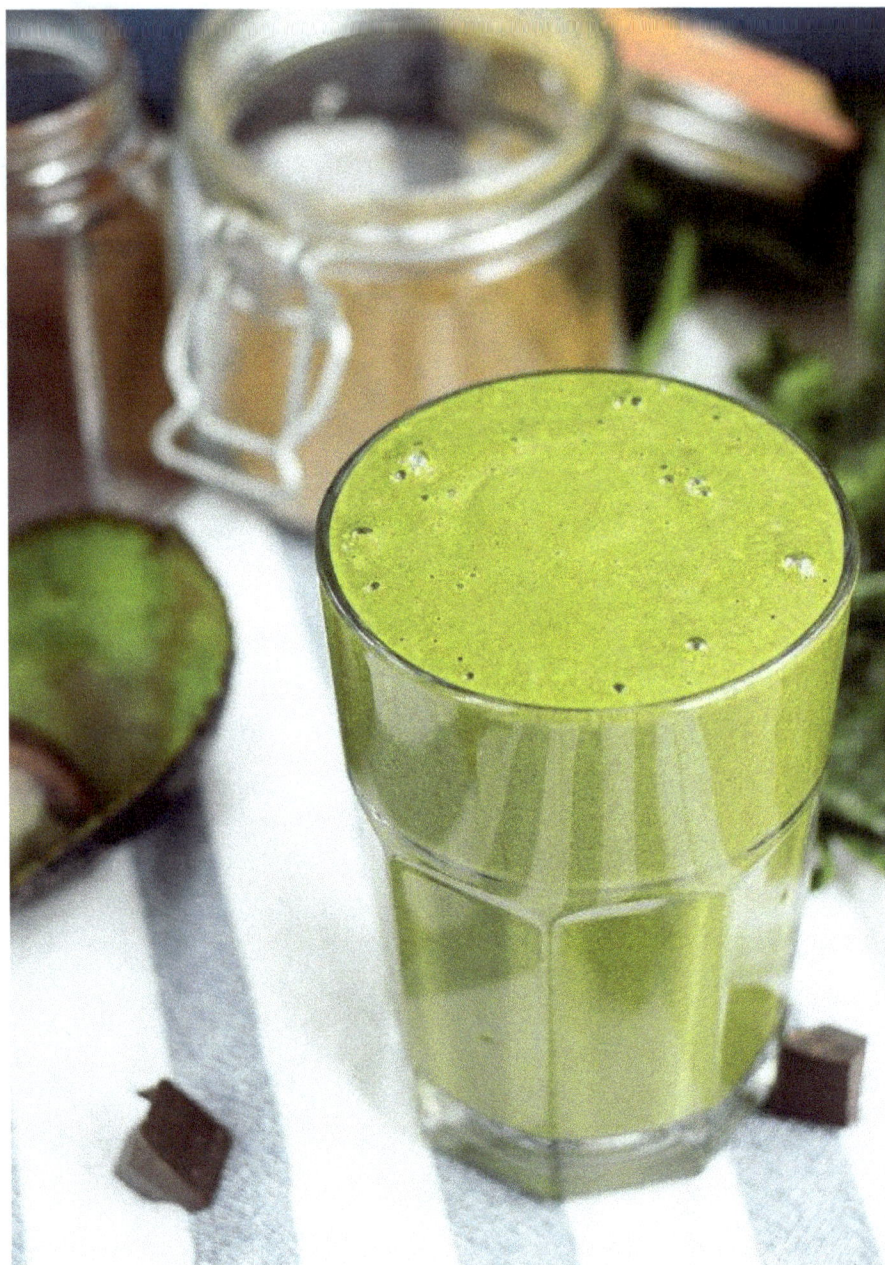

Preparation Time: 10 minutes

Cooking Time: 0 minutes

Servings: 2

Ingredients :

- 2 cups fresh baby spinach
- ½ avocado, peeled, pitted, and chopped
- 4-6 drops liquid stevia
- ½ teaspoon ground cinnamon
- 1 tablespoon hemp seeds
- 2 cups chilled alkaline water

Directions:

1. Add all the Ingredients in a high-speed blender and pulse until smooth.

2. Pour the smoothie into two glasses and serve immediately.

Nutrition:

Calories 132

Total Fat 11.7 g

Saturated Fat 2.2 g

Cholesterol 0 mg

Sodium 27 mg

Total Carbs 6.1 g

Fiber 4.5 g

Sugar 0.4 g

Protein 3.1 g

Dandelion Avocado Smoothie

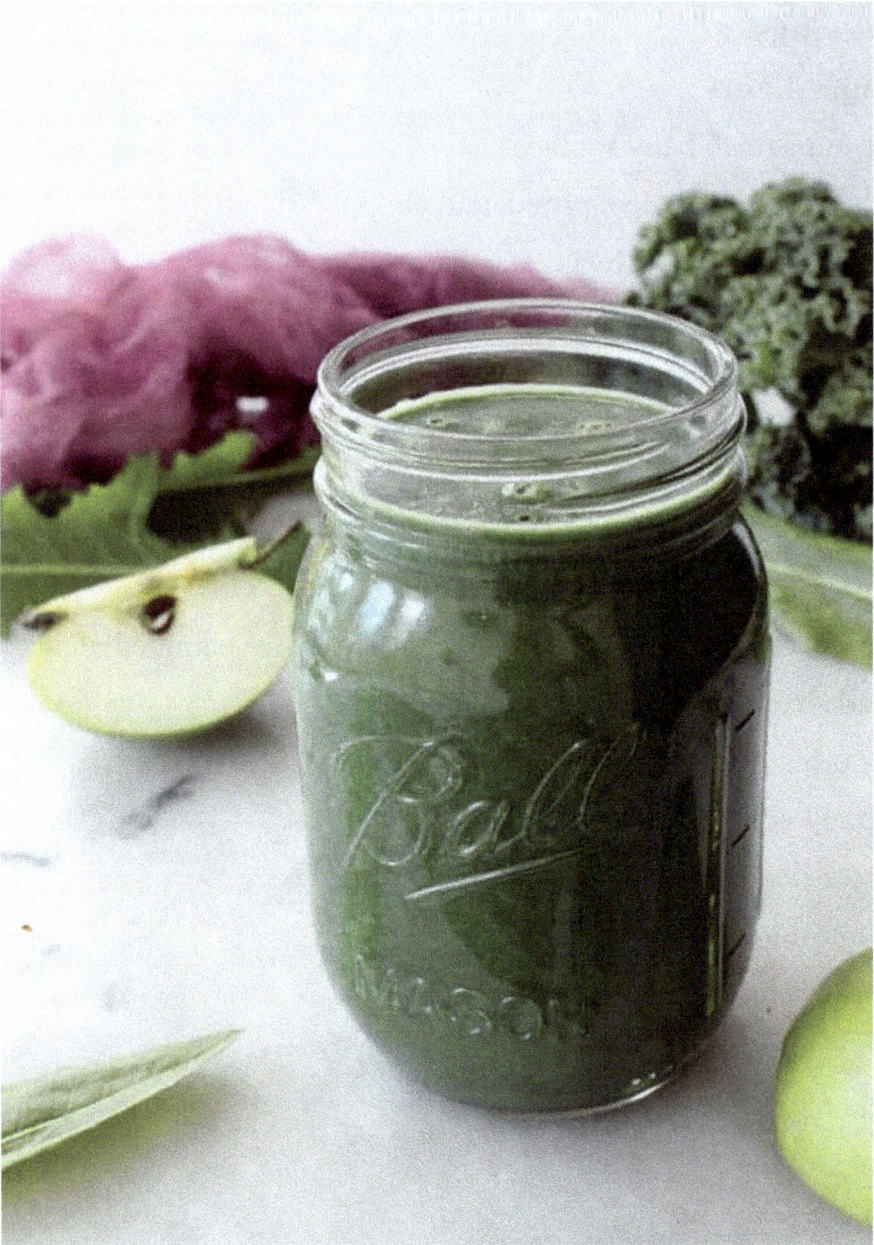

Preparation Time: 15 minutes

Cooking Time: 0

Servings: 1

Ingredients :

• One cup of Dandelion

• One Orange (juiced)

• Coconut water

• One Avocado

• One key lime (juice)

Directions:

1. In a high-speed blender until smooth, blend **Ingredients** .

Nutrition:

Calories: 160

Fat: 15 grams

Carbohydrates: 9 grams

Protein: 2 grams

Amaranth Greens And Avocado Smoothie

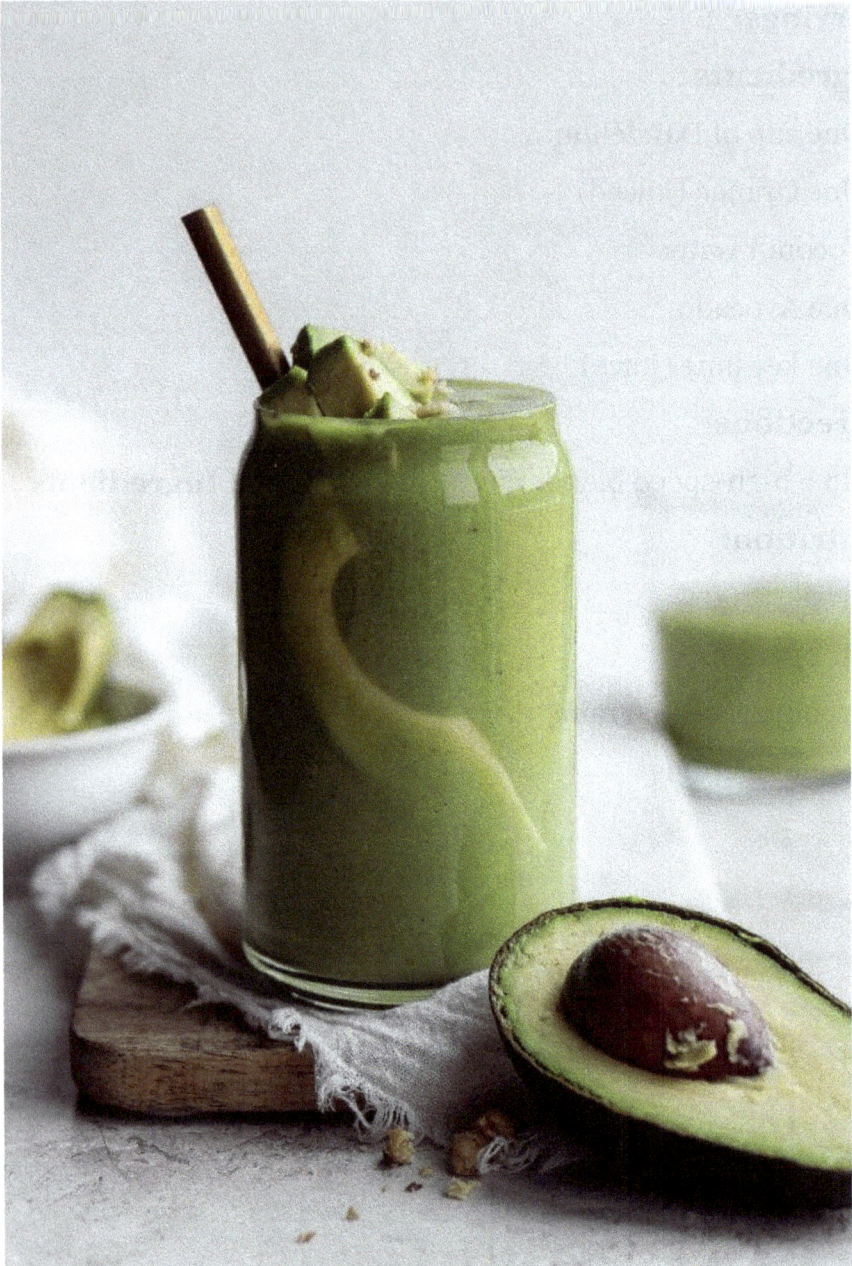

Preparation Time: 15 minutes

Cooking Time: 0

Servings: 1

Ingredients :

• One key lime (juice).

• Two sliced apples (seeded).

• Half avocado.

• Two cupsful of amaranth greens.

• Two cupsful of watercress.

• One cupful of water.

Directions:

1. Add the whole recipes together and transfer them into the blender. Blend thoroughly until smooth.

Nutrition:

Calories: 160

Fat: 15 grams

Carbohydrates: 9 grams

Protein: 2 grams

Lettuce, Orange And Banana Smoothie

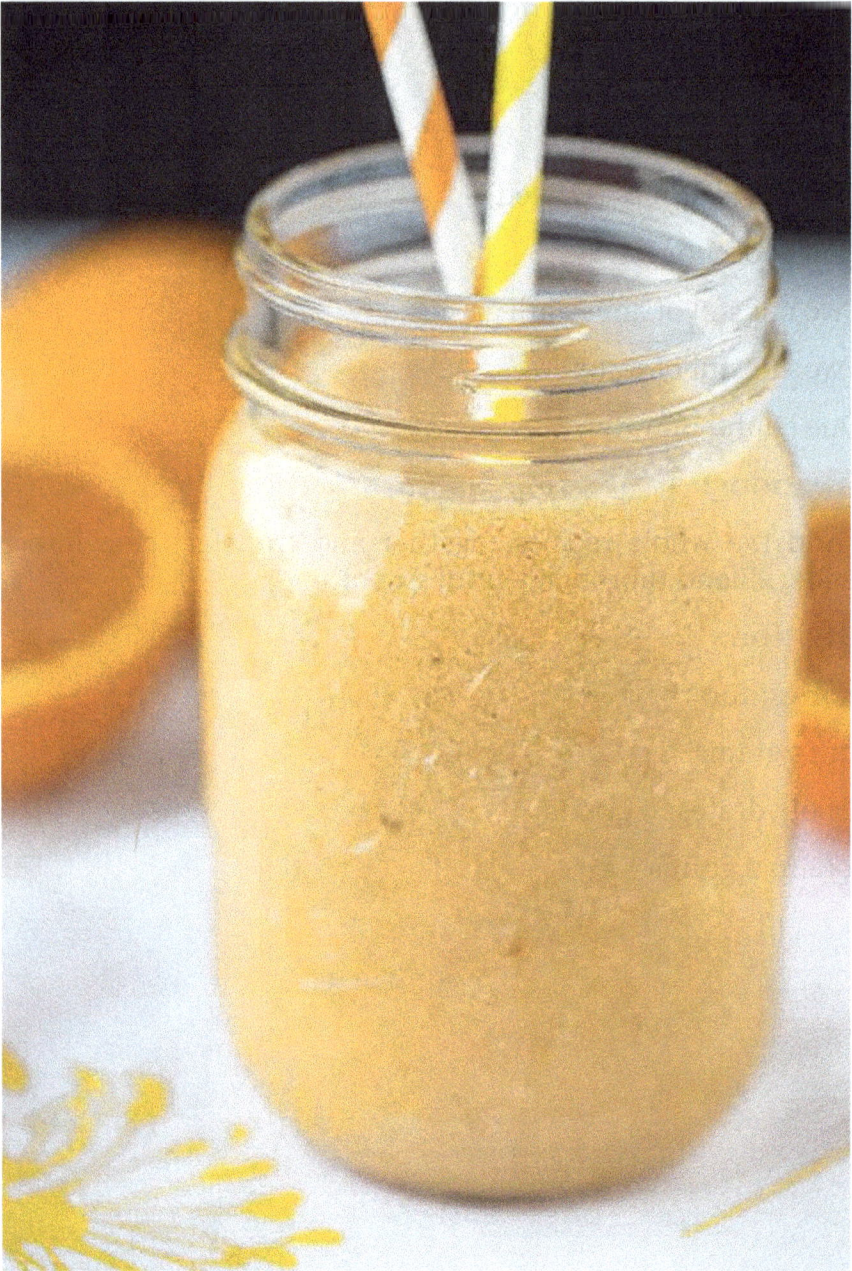

Preparation Time: 15 minutes

Cooking Time: 0

Servings: 1

Ingredients :

• One and a half cupsful of fresh lettuce.

• One large banana.

• One cup of mixed berries of your choice.

• One juiced orange.

Directions:

1. First, add the orange juice to your blender.

2. Add the remaining recipes and blend thoroughly.

3. Enjoy the rest of your day.

Nutrition:

Calories: 252.1

Protein: 4.1 g

Delicious Elderberry Smoothie

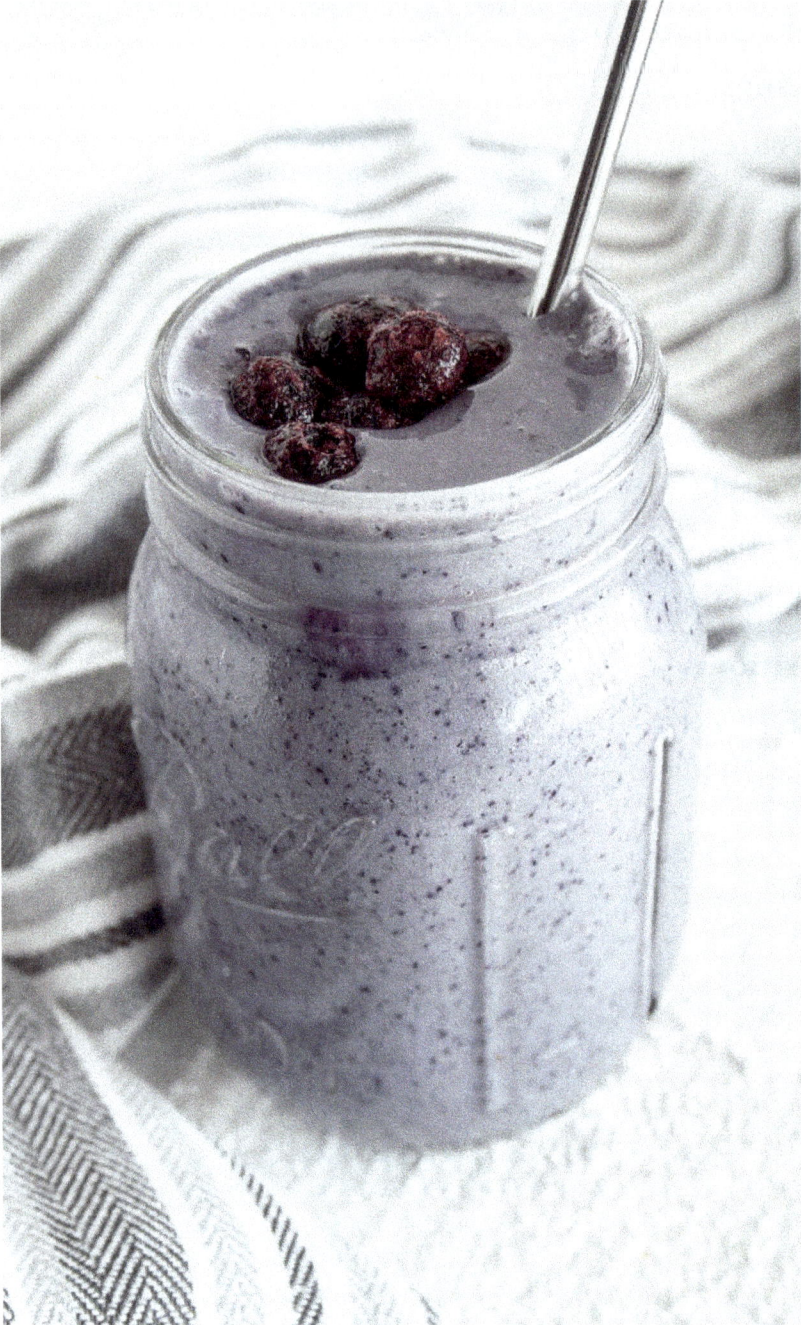

Preparation Time: 15 minutes

Cooking Time: 0

Servings: 1

Ingredients :

- One cupful of Elderberry

- One cupful of Cucumber

- One large apple

- A quarter cupful of water

Directions:

1. Add the whole recipes together into a blender. Grind very well until they are uniformly smooth and enjoy.

Nutrition:

Calories: 106

Carbohydrates: 26.68

Peaches Zucchini Smoothie

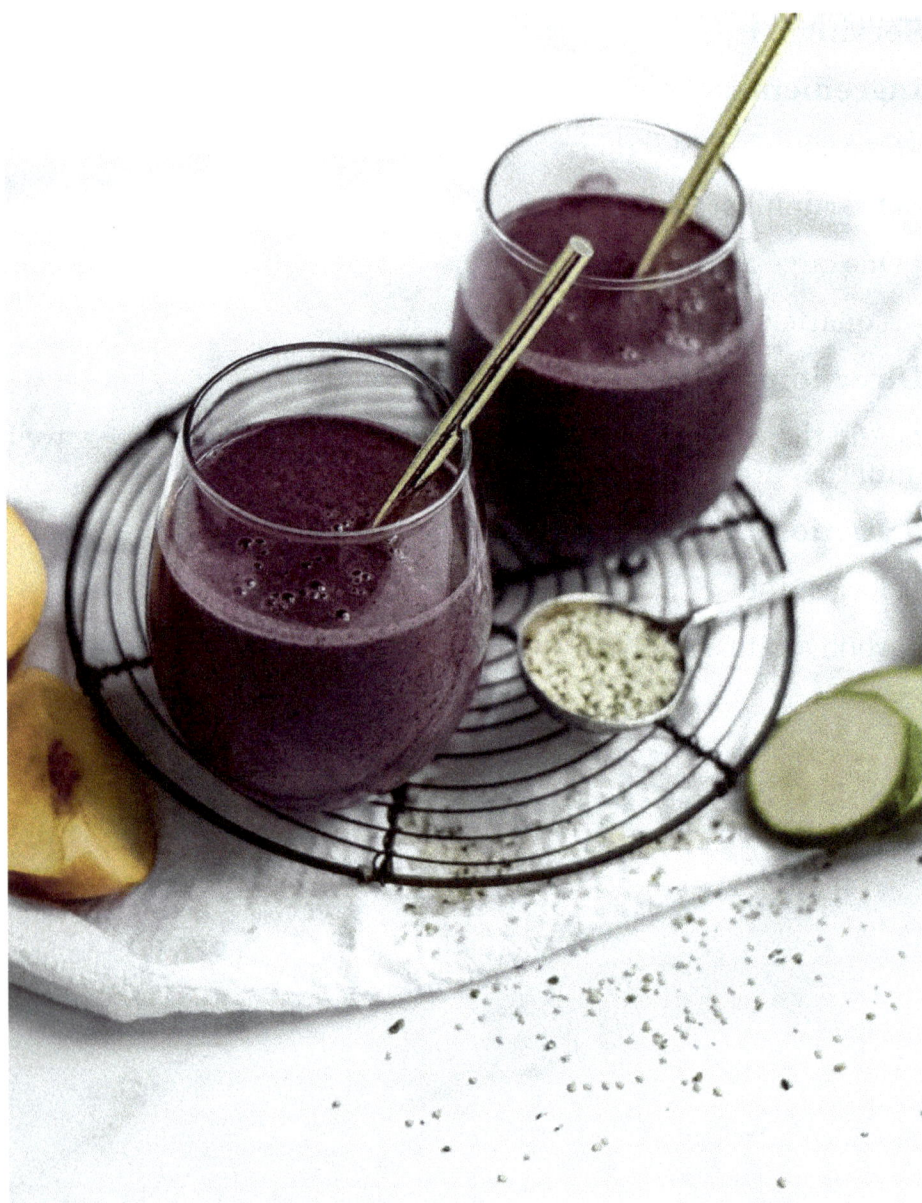

Preparation Time: 15 minutes

Cooking Time: 0

Servings: 1

Ingredients :

• A half cupful of squash.

• A half cupful of peaches.

• A quarter cupful of coconut water.

• A half cupful of Zucchini.

Directions:

1. Add the whole recipes together into a blender and blend until smooth and serve.

Nutrition:

55 Calories

0g Fat

2g Of Protein

10mg Sodium

14 G Carbohydrate

2g Of Fiber

Ginger Orange And Strawberry Smoothie

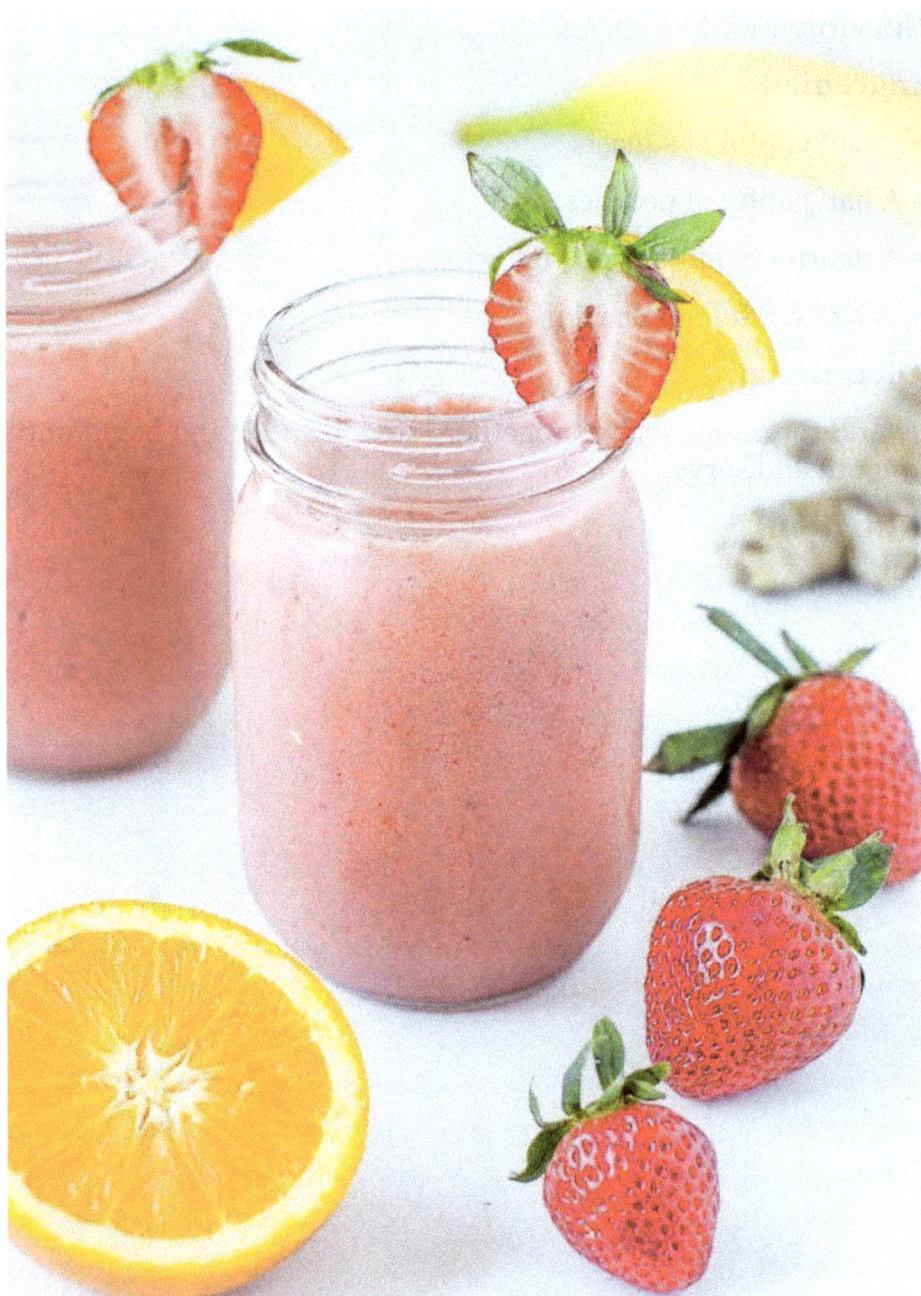

Preparation Time: 15 minutes

Cooking Time: 0

Servings: 1

Ingredients :

• One cup of strawberry.

• One large orange (juice)

• One large banana.

• Quarter small sized ginger (peeled and sliced).

Directions:

2. Transfer the orange juice to a clean blender.

3. Add the remaining recipes and blend thoroughly until smooth.

4. Enjoy. Wow! You have ended the 9th day of your weight loss and detox journey.

Nutrition:

32 Calories

0.3g Fat

2g Of Protein

10mg Sodium

14g Carbohydrate

Water

2g Of Fiber.

Kale Parsley And Chia Seeds Detox Smoothie

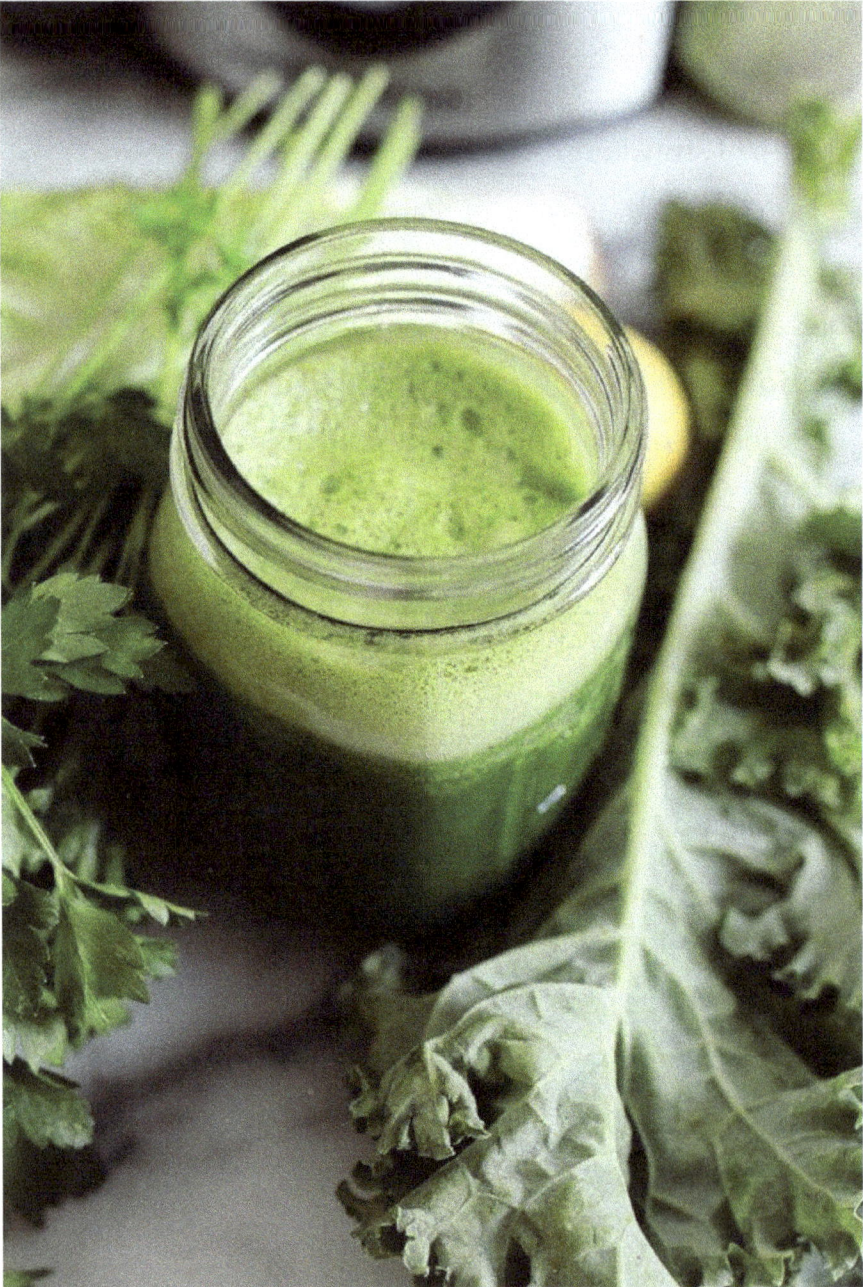

Preparation Time: 15 minutes

Cooking Time: 0

Servings: 1

Ingredients :

• Three tbsp. chia seeds (grounded).

• One cupful of water.

• One sliced banana.

• One pear (chopped).

• One cupful of organic kale.

• One cupful of parsley.

• Two tbsp. of lemon juice.

• A dash of cinnamon.

Directions:

1. Add the whole recipes together into a blender and pour the water before blending. Blend at high speed until smooth and enjoy. You may or may not place it in the refrigerator depending on how hot or cold the weather appears.

Nutrition:

75 calories

1g fat

5g protein

10g fibre

Watermelon Limenade

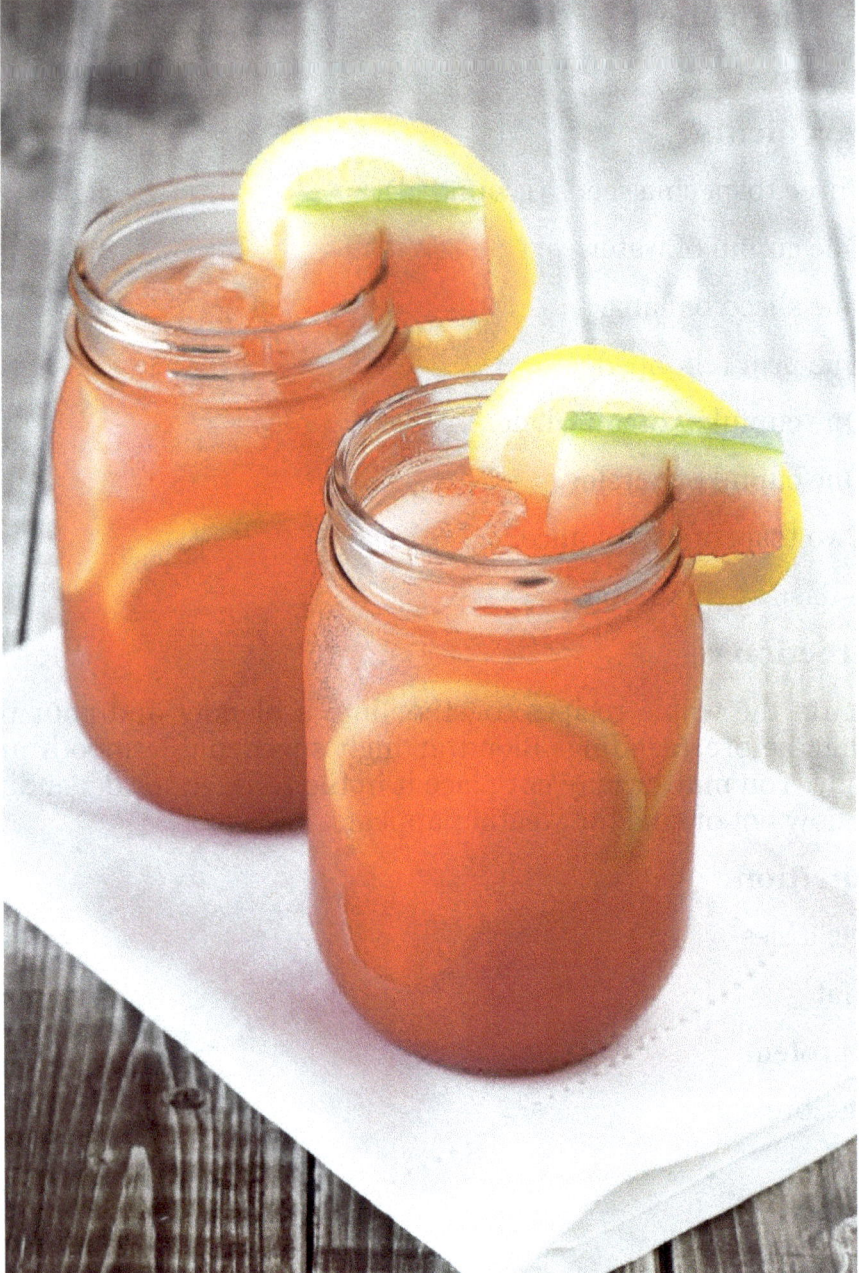

Preparation Time: 5 Minutes

Cooking Time: 0 minutes

Servings: 6

When it comes to refreshing summertime drinks, lemonade is always near the top of the list. This Watermelon "Limenade" is perfect for using up leftover watermelon or for those early fall days when stores and farmers are almost giving them away. You can also substitute 4 cups of ice for the cold water to create a delicious summertime slushy.

Ingredients

- 4 cups diced watermelon

- 4 cups cold water

- 2 tablespoons freshly squeezed lemon juice

- 1 tablespoon freshly squeezed lime juice

Directions:

1. In a blender, combine the watermelon, water, lemon juice, and lime juice, and blend for 1 minute.

2. Strain the contents through a fine-mesh sieve or nut-milk bag. Serve chilled. Store in the refrigerator for up to 3 days.

SERVING TIP: Slice up a few lemon or lime wedges to serve with your Watermelon Limenade, or top it with a few fresh mint leaves to give it an extra-crisp, minty flavor.

Nutrition:

Calories: 60

Bubbly Orange Soda

Preparation Time: 5 Minutes

Cooking Time: 0 minutes

Servings: 4

Soda can be one of the toughest things to give up when you first adopt a WFPB diet. That's partially because refined sugars and caffeine are addictive, but it can also be because carbonated beverages are fun to drink! With sweetness from the orange juice and bubbliness from the carbonated water, this orange "soda" is perfect for assisting in the transition from SAD to WFPB.

Ingredients

• 4 cups carbonated water

• 2 cups pulp-free orange juice (4 oranges, freshly squeezed and strained)

Directions:

1. For each serving, pour 2 parts carbonated water and 1-part orange juice over ice right before serving.

2. Stir and enjoy.

SERVING TIP: This recipe is best made right before drinking. The amount of fizz in the carbonated water will decrease the longer it's open, so if you're going to make it ahead of time, make sure it's stored in an airtight, refrigerator-safe container.

Nutrition:

Calories: 56

Creamy Cashew Milk

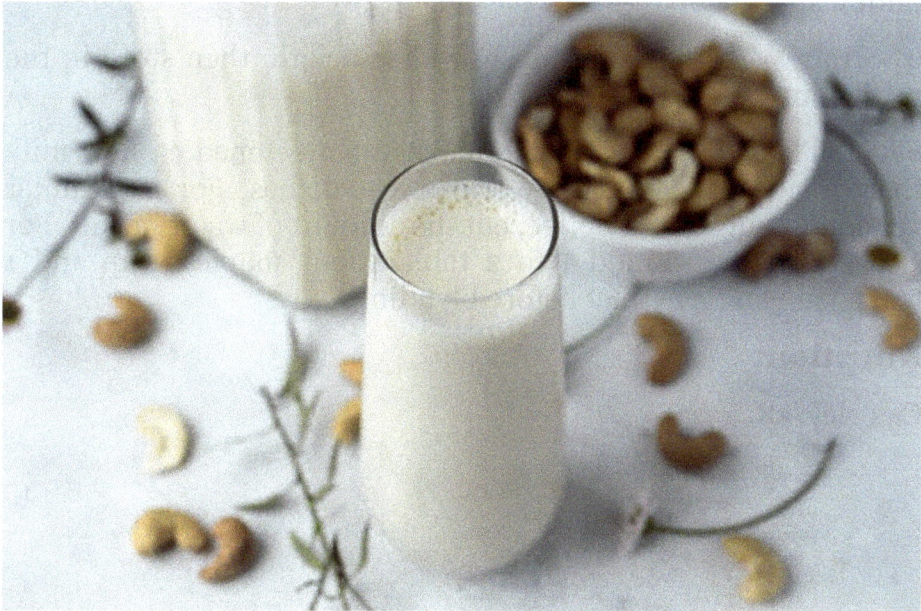

Preparation Time: 5 Minutes

Cooking Time: 0 minutes

Servings: 8

Learning how to make your own plant-based milks can be one of the best ways to save money and ditch dairy for good. This is one of the easiest milk recipes to master, and if you have a high-speed blender, you can skip the straining step and go straight to a refrigerator-safe container. Large mason jars work great for storing plant-based milk, as they allow you to give a quick shake before each use.

Ingredients

• 4 cups water

• ¼ cup raw cashews, soaked overnight

Directions:

1. In a blender, blend the water and cashews on high speed for 2 minutes.

2. Strain with a nut-milk bag or cheesecloth, then store in the refrigerator for up to 5 days.

VARIATION TIP: This recipe makes unsweetened cashew milk that can be used in savory and sweet dishes. For a creamier version to put in your coffee, cut the amount of water in half. For a sweeter version, add 1 to 2 tablespoons maple syrup and 1 teaspoon vanilla extract before blending.

Nutrition:

Calories: 18

Homemade Oat Milk

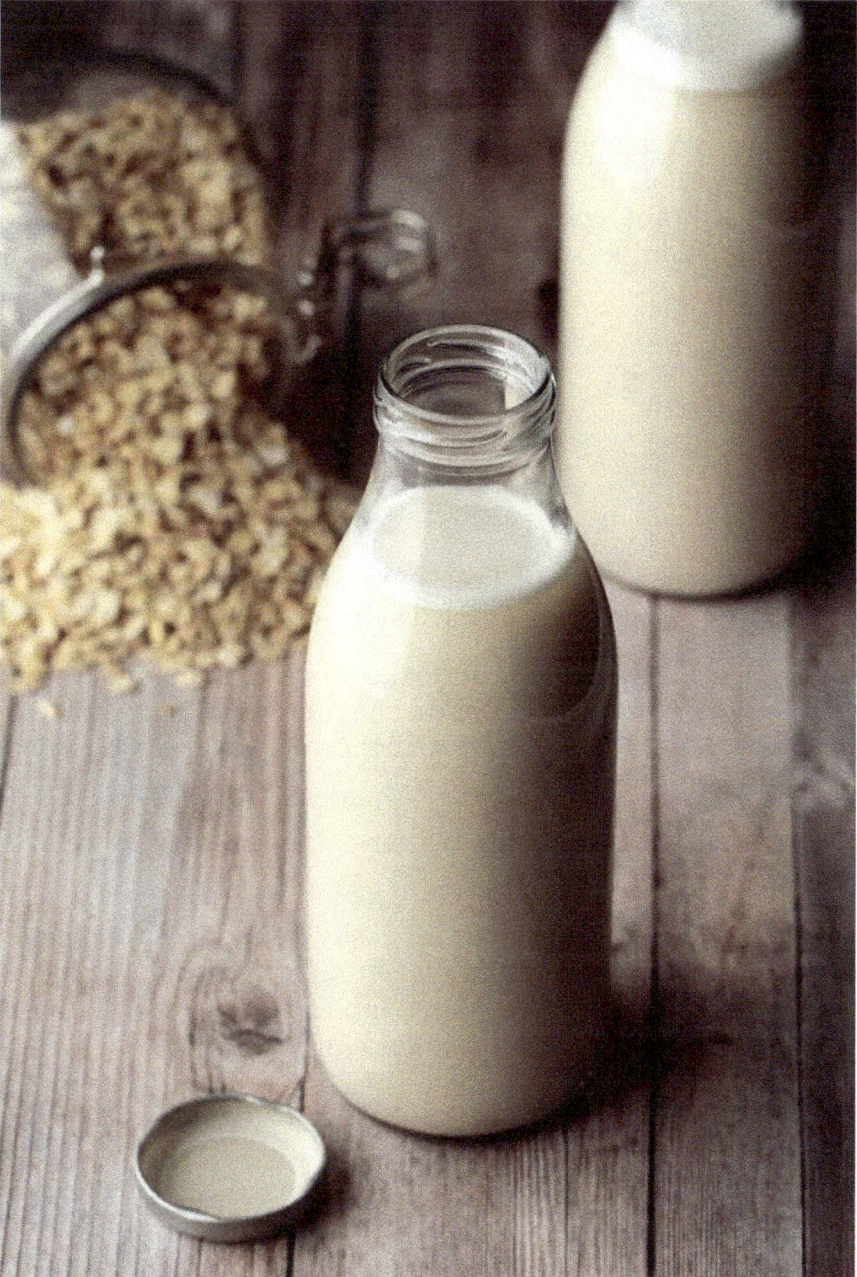

Preparation Time: 5 Minutes

Cooking Time: 0 minutes

Servings: 8

Oat milk is a fantastic option if you need a nut-free milk or just want an extremely inexpensive plant-based milk. Making a half-gallon jar at home costs a fraction of the price of other plant-based or dairy milks. Oat milk can be used in both savory and sweet dishes.

Ingredients

• 1 cup rolled oats

• 4 cups water

Directions:

1. Put the oats in a medium bowl, and cover with cold water. Soak for 15 minutes, then drain and rinse the oats.

2. Pour the cold water and the soaked oats into a blender. Blend for 60 to 90 seconds, or just until the mixture is a creamy white color throughout. (Blending any further may overblend the oats, resulting in a gummy milk.)

3. Strain through a nut-milk bag or colander, then store in the refrigerator for up to 5 days.

VARIATION TIP: This recipe can easily be made into chocolate oat milk. Once you've strained the oat milk, return it to a blender with 3 tablespoons cocoa powder, 2 tablespoons maple syrup, and 1 teaspoon vanilla extract, then blend for 30 seconds.

Nutrition:

Calories: 39

Lucky Mint Smoothie

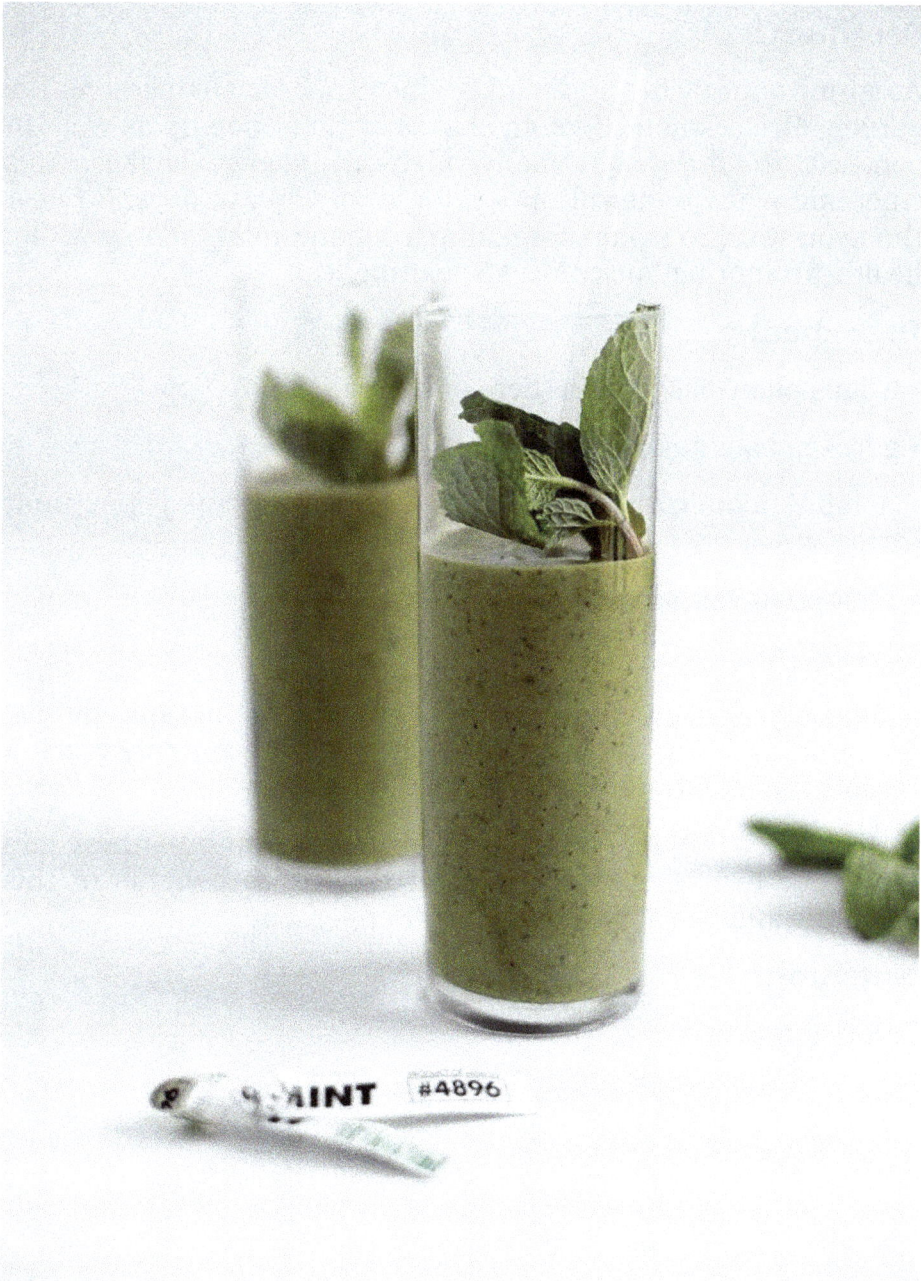

Preparation Time: 5 Minutes

Cooking Time: 0 minutes

Servings: 2

As spring approaches and mint begins to once again take over the garden, "Irish"-themed green shakes begin to pop up as well. In contrast to the traditionally high-fat, sugary shakes, this smoothie is a wonderful option for sunny spring days. So next time you want to sip on something cool and minty, do so with a health-promoting Lucky Mint Smoothie.

Ingredients

• 2 cups plant-based milk (here or here)

• 2 frozen bananas, halved

• 1 tablespoon fresh mint leaves or ¼ teaspoon peppermint extract

• 1 teaspoon vanilla extract

Directions:

1. In a blender, combine the milk, bananas, mint, and vanilla. Blend on high for 1 to 2 minutes, or until the contents reach a smooth and creamy consistency, and serve.

VARIATION TIP: If you like to sneak greens into smoothies, add a cup or two of spinach to boost the health benefits of this smoothie and give it an even greener appearance.

Nutrition:

Calories: 152

Paradise Island Smoothie

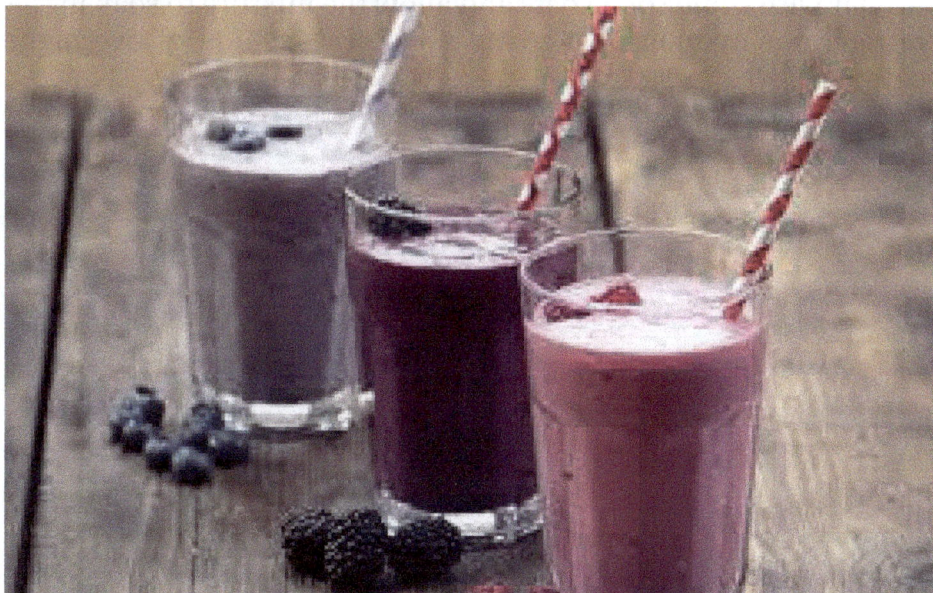

Preparation Time: 5 Minutes

Cooking Time: 0 minutes

Servings: 2

Ingredients :

- 2 cups plant-based milk (here or here)
- 1 frozen banana
- ½ cup frozen mango chunks
- ½ cup frozen pineapple chunks
- 1 teaspoon vanilla extract

Directions:

1. In a blender, combine the milk, banana, mango, pineapple, and vanilla. Blend on high for 1 to 2 minutes, or until the contents reach a smooth and creamy consistency, and serve.

LEFTOVER TIP: If you have any leftover smoothie, you can put it in a jar with some rolled oats and allow the mixture to soak in the refrigerator overnight to create a tropical version of overnight oats.

Nutrition:

Calories: 176

Apple Pie Smoothie

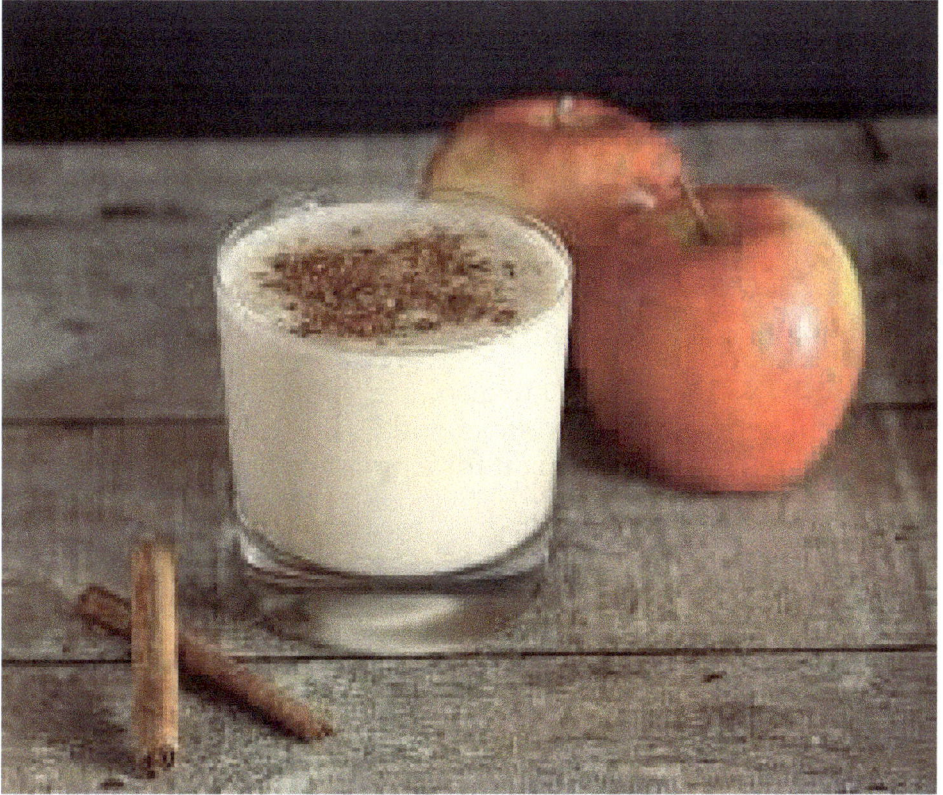

Preparation Time: 5 Minutes

Cooking Time: 0 minutes

Servings: 2

This smoothie is great for a quick breakfast or a cool dessert. Its combination of sweet apples and warming cinnamon is sure to win over children and adults alike. If the holidays find you in a warm area, this smoothie may just be the cool treat you've been looking for to take the place of pie at dessert time.

Ingredients

• 2 sweet crisp apples, cut into 1-inch cubes

• 2 cups plant-based milk (here or here)

- 1 cup ice

- 1 tablespoon maple syrup

- 1 teaspoon ground cinnamon

- 1 teaspoon vanilla extract

Directions:

1. In a blender, combine the apples, milk, ice, maple syrup, cinnamon, and vanilla. Blend on high for 1 to 2 minutes, or until the contents reach a smooth and creamy consistency, and serve.

VARIATION TIP: You can also use this recipe for making overnight oatmeal. Blend your smoothie, mix it with 2 cups rolled oats, and refrigerate overnight for a premade breakfast for two.

Nutrition:

Calories: 198